THE PICKER/COMMONWEALTH PROGRAM FOR PATIENT-CENTERED CARE

The Picker/Commonwealth Program for Patient-Centered Care was established in 1987 at Boston's Beth Israel Hospital and the Harvard Medical School to promote an approach to hospital and health services focusing on the patient's needs and concerns, as the patient defines them, and to explore models of care that make the experience of illness and hospitalization more humane. The program defines seven dimensions of patient-centered care in the inpatient setting:

1. Respect for patients' values, preferences, and expressed needs
2. Coordination and integration of care
3. Information, communication, and education
4. Physical comfort
5. Emotional support and alleviation of fear and anxiety
6. Involvement of family and friends
7. Transition and continuity

To assess patients' experiences within these dimensions, the program has developed a distinct survey instrument designed to elicit *reports* from patients about concrete aspects of their experience, in lieu of the *ratings* of satisfaction generally called for on patient surveys. Using this instrument in 1989 to gauge the status of patient-centered care in U.S. hospitals, the program surveyed over 6,400 recent hospital patients, randomly selected from sixty-two hospitals nationwide, along with 2,000 of the friends or family members who served as their care partners. Any hospital wishing to do so may now purchase patient-survey services using the Picker/Commonwealth instrument.

Since its inception, the program has become a central resource for information, technical assistance, and consultative services. The program's newsletter, *Picker/Commonwealth Report*, reaches over 4,000 individuals and institutions with information about patient-centered innovations and programs.

The work of the Picker/Commonwealth Program has also generated a momentum that is carrying the concept of patient-centered care into other arenas of health care. Program staff currently collaborate with task forces of hospital directors working on the practical uses of patient survey data to identify unmet needs, promote patient-centered care, stimulate organizational change, and incorporate feedback from patients into ongoing quality-monitoring systems. As the burden of acute care shifts away from inpatient settings, program staff also work with several professional organizations—including the American College of Physicians, the National Association of Community Health Centers, and an association of group-practice health maintenance organizations—to adapt the survey instrument and apply the principles of patient-centered care to the outpatient arena.

In addition, program activity has stimulated interest in the concept of patient-centered care and its assessment in foreign countries. Colleagues in Canada, the United Kingdom, and Germany are adapting the Picker/Commonwealth survey instrument to conduct national patient surveys in those countries.

For additional information, contact

The Picker/Commonwealth Program
for Patient-Centered Care
Beth Israel Hospital
330 Brookline Avenue
Boston, Massachusetts 02215-5491
(617) 735-2388
FAX (617) 735-2854

Through
the Patient's
Eyes

MARGARET GERTEIS
SUSAN EDGMAN-LEVITAN
JENNIFER DALEY
THOMAS L. DELBANCO
EDITORS

Through the Patient's Eyes

Understanding and Promoting Patient-Centered Care

Jossey-Bass Publishers · San Francisco

Substantial discounts on bulk quantities of Jossey-Bass books are available to corporations, professional associations, and other organizations. For details and discount information, contact the special sales department at Jossey-Bass Inc., Publishers. (415) 433-1740; Fax (415) 433-0499.

For sales outside the United States, contact Maxwell Macmillan International Publishing Group, 866 Third Avenue, New York, New York 10022.

Manufactured in the United States of America

 The paper used in this book is acid-free and meets the State of California requirements for recycled paper (50 percent recycled waste, including 10 percent postconsumer waste), which are the strictest guidelines for recycled paper currently in use in the United States.

Portions of an article by Thomas W. Moloney and Barbara Paul, "The Consumer Movement Takes Hold in Medical Care," *Health Affairs, 10,* 1991, pp. 268–278, are reprinted with permission in Chapter Twelve.

Library of Congress Cataloging-in-Publication Data

Through the patient's eyes : understanding and promoting patient-centered care / editors, Margaret Gerteis, Susan Edgman-Levitan, Jennifer Daley, and associates. — 1st ed.
    p.   cm. — (The Jossey-Bass health series)
  Includes bibliographical references and index.
  ISBN 1-55542-544-5 (alk. paper)
  1. Physician and patient. I. Gerteis, Margaret. II. Edgman-Levitan, Susan. III. Daley, Jennifer. IV. Series.
  [DNLM: 1. Patient Care Planning. 2. Patient Satisfaction.
3. Professional-Patient Relations.   W 84.7 T531 1993]
R727.3.T5   1993
610.69'6—dc20
DNLM/DLC
for Library of Congress   93-51
                                     CIP

FIRST EDITION
HB Printing   10 9 8 7 6 5 4 3 2   *Code 9347*

THE JOSSEY-BASS HEALTH SERIES

CONTENTS

PREFACE

Quality—the catchphrase of the 1990s in health and medical care—
has two dimensions. One has to do with technical excellence: the
skill and competence of professionals and the ability of diagnostic
or therapeutic equipment, procedures, and systems to accomplish
what they are meant to accomplish, reliably and effectively. Borrowing the language and conceptual models of industrial engineering,
we speak in this sense of "quality control," "quality assurance,"
and "quality improvement."

The other dimension relates to subjective experience—its texture and substance, its sentient quality. In this sense, we speak of
the quality of a sensation or experience or the quality of human
relationships. In health care, it is quality in this subjective dimension that patients experience most directly—in their perception of
illness or well-being and in their encounters with health care professionals and institutions.

This is not a book about health care quality in the first,
technical sense—although the health care system unquestionably
stands to benefit from the attention that subject attracts today. This
is a book about quality in the second sense—the experience of illness and health care *through the patient's eyes.* Health care professionals and decision makers are uneasy about addressing this "soft"
subject, given the hard, intractable, and unyielding problems of
financing, access, and clinical effectiveness in health care. But the

experiential dimension of quality is not trivial. It is the heart of what patients want from health care—enhancement of their sense of well-being, relief from their suffering. *Any* health care system, however it may be financed or structured, must address both aspects of quality to achieve legitimacy in the eyes of those it serves.

The Picker/Commonwealth Program for Patient-Centered Care was established in 1987, with financial support from The Commonwealth Fund of New York, to explore patients' needs and concerns, as patients themselves define them, and to promote models of care that make the experience of illness and hospitalization more humane. To begin, we conducted focus groups with patients and their family members, reviewed the literature, and consulted with health care professionals. On the basis of what we read and heard, we defined seven dimensions of patient-centered care, including (1) respect for patients' values, preferences, and expressed needs; (2) coordination and integration of care; (3) information, communication, and education; (4) physical comfort; (5) emotional support and alleviation of fear and anxiety; (6) involvement of family and friends; and (7) transition and continuity. Program consultants, using a survey instrument designed to elicit reports from patients about concrete aspects of their experience within these dimensions, then interviewed over 6,000 recently hospitalized patients, randomly selected from sixty-two hospitals nationwide, along with 2,000 of the friends or family members who served as their care partners. Program staff and consultants also visited more than twenty hospitals, including those identified as exemplary by experts in the field and hospitals that scored high or low on the national survey. In the pages that follow, we offer the preliminary results of these inquiries.

We stake no exclusive claim to the territory explored in these pages, nor do we pretend to be lone pioneers. Virtually everyone who works in health care is motivated by an honest desire to help people, and many different and well-established professional perspectives inform this work. Doctors and medical ethicists have long recognized and struggled with the dilemmas that arise when patients' values conflict with those of clinicians. The nursing profession in particular contributes to every dimension of patient-centered care, working to enhance the personal aspects of caring and serving often as the personal link between patients and a seemingly impersonal institution. Social workers understand the larger social context of illness and its implications for treatment and recovery. Organizational theorists and management consultants help identify many of the structural and operational barriers to customer service and patient-centered quality. We cannot hope to do justice in this volume to the richness of these and other professional contributions, although we do try to acknowledge them wherever appropriate.

There is nevertheless an important difference between these perspectives and ours. Each professional group is shaped by its own unique history, ideology, and professional agenda. Our conscious effort throughout this project, however, has been to set aside these *professional* frames of reference in order to cast a clearer light on the *patient's* perspective. We invite the reader, at least for the time being, to do the same. Our aim is to find out what patients want, need, and experience in health care, not what professionals (however well-motivated) believe they need or get. And yet it is not an easy task for any of us to confront the boundaries of our own preconceptions, as we have discovered time and again over the past five years. Moreover, health care providers must respond to many other legitimate constraints, pressures, and concerns—organizational, financial, political, professional, personal, and regulatory. We try, too, to acknowledge these other realities throughout this book, but they are not our central focus. It is not our purpose here, for example, to help hospitals find ways to avoid uncompensated days of care—although this concern may motivate many to improve their educational efforts or to better manage the transition to home, both of which may also serve the patient's interests. What we hope to accomplish, rather, is to help health care providers keep the patient's perspective in mind as they respond to the pressures of the "real" world.

Audience

The concept of patient-centered care provides a common ground for patients worried about their health and well-being, managers worried about competition and efficiency, clinicians worried about quality of care, and payers worried about cost-effectiveness to talk and work together. We write primarily with the administrators and senior managers of hospitals and health care facilities in mind, to whom we offer a framework for thinking about, assessing, and managing the quality of care from the patient's perspective. But those responsible for clinical care who may be skeptical of service-quality programs designed principally for marketing purposes will find an approach firmly grounded in the best traditions of clinical practice here. For department heads and middle managers—key players in the success of any patient-centered organizational strategy—this book further offers both a structured way to reexamine their own areas of responsibility and practical approaches to improving the services under their charge. Ultimately, the task of creating humane, equitable, high-quality health care will fall to everyone who works in the field—especially to those record numbers of students now preparing for careers in health care. They, too, will benefit from examining health care services and institutions through the patient's eyes. Finally, we address health regulators and policy makers who, we hope, will find here both a stimulus and a preliminary framework for incorporating the patient's perspective into ongoing quality standards and monitoring systems.

The information gathered for this project—from the literature, focus groups, informal meetings and discussions, national survey, and field visits—and the insights gained as a result provide the material for this book. We have set out to address three principal questions: How do patients' interactions with health care providers, institutions, and systems affect their subjective experience of illness and well-being? How do those systems work, and fail to work, to meet patients' needs? How can health care providers, managers, and planners incorporate the patient's perspective to improve health care quality?

Overview of the Contents

In the introductory chapter, we set the stage by describing the patient's perspective on health care, why it matters, and why it is so often overlooked, and we explain in greater detail the "dimensions of patient-centered care" that provide the conceptual framework for our work.

The chapters in Part One (Chapters Two through Nine)

summarize what we have learned through our inquiries, dimension by dimension. Each chapter provides a structure for thinking about quality from the patient's perspective within that dimension, explores the problems that patients typically encounter and the causes of those problems, and suggests practical approaches to solving them. A summary of the major points covered and a list of suggestions for improving the quality of care are provided at the end of each chapter.

In Chapter Two, Kimberly D. Allshouse focuses on the broad aspects of respecting patients' individuality: understanding how their cultural beliefs, values, and practices affect their perceptions of illness and expectations for treatment; eliciting and respecting their preferences for involvement in clinical care; and elucidating patients' therapeutic goals and weighing appropriate treatment options.

Margaret Gerteis examines factors that affect patients' perceptions of the competence and efficiency of their caregivers in Chapter Three. She focuses on three distinct tasks of coordination unique to the environment of hospitals and health care facilities: 1) coordination of clinical care, across specialties and professional hierarchies; 2) coordination of diagnostic and therapeutic clinical support services; and 3) coordination of the delivery of nursing and ancillary "front-line" patient care.

In Chapter Four, Jennifer Daley discusses, from the patient's perspective, some of the issues in communication that may arise between patients and their caregivers (physicians and nurses) and describes some innovative interventions that have proved helpful.

Beth Ellers examines the components of a patient-centered approach to education in Chapter Five and discusses intervention strategies and programs that can improve the quality of patient-centered education in an institutional setting.

In Chapter Six, Janice D. Walker focuses on the basic task of minimizing physical trauma during the acute phase of illness and maximizing comfort and healing in the recovery phase. She addresses three principal aspects of this task: controlling acute pain, providing care to support and maintain normal body functions, and minimizing the stresses of the hospital's physical environment to provide a supportive atmosphere for healing and recovery.

Susan Edgman-Levitan, in Chapter Seven, explores issues relating to patients' needs for social and emotional support and describes, from the patient's perspective, approaches that health care institutions can use to provide such support, ranging from simple techniques designed to bolster self-esteem to more sophisticated programs.

In Chapter Eight, Beth Ellers explores the functions families serve and the realities they face in their role as caregivers or care partners, as long-term promoters of health and well-being, and as providers of essential social and emotional support. She examines the issues of family involvement from the distinct but overlapping, and sometimes conflicting, perspectives of patient, family, and provider and reviews programs and interventions that help health care institutions accommodate families.

In Chapter Nine, Beth Ellers and Janice D. Walker examine the issues patients and their families face when they move out of the institutional setting of health care and they suggest ways that health care providers can help ease the transition and promote continuity of care.

The three chapters in Part Two are structured as essays with a broader focus, addressing questions about patient-centered care and the larger environment of health care that arise repeatedly in our work—namely, What makes some hospitals more patient-centered than others? How can we get doctors more involved? and How does patient-centeredness fit in with health care policy, standards, and regulation?

In Chapter Ten, Margaret Gerteis and Marc J. Roberts take a look at the larger environment of the institutions themselves. Using the results of the national survey of hospital patients to "map" the institutional landscape of patient-centered care, they examine the characteristics that make hospitals patient-centered and their practical implications for managers trying to create more patient-centered institutions.

In Chapter Eleven, Thomas L. Delbanco explores "through the patient's eyes" the role doctors play and proposes strategies to involve doctors more actively in improving patients' experiences with hospital care.

In the final chapter (Chapter Twelve), Thomas W. Moloney

and Barbara Paul discuss the current crisis of public confidence and
the need to restore public faith in the medical system. They review
the social, demographic, and technological forces that are fueling
a growing demand for a more patient-responsive system and examine the emerging patient-centered science of care that promises to
help bridge the gulf between patients and practitioners and rebuild
public trust and confidence.

Acknowledgments

This book is very much the product of the Picker/Commonwealth
Program for Patient-Centered Care. The credit for whatever contribution it makes to health care in this country must first go to
Harvey and Jean Picker, whose gift to The Commonwealth Fund
provided the opportunity to explore and promote the humane aspects of medical care. As Margaret E. Mahoney, president of the
fund, recently observed of the Pickers, "It is suggestive of their
insight and sagacity that the family that quite literally built the
academic base for the science of radiology should recognize an equal
imperative to understand medical care from the patient's perspective." Jean Picker, sadly, died in 1990; Harvey Picker has continued
to be an inspiration and a sage counsel to the program that bears
his name.

The directors and officers of The Commonwealth Fund have
been unfailing in their support and constructive in their criticism
throughout the program's history. Margaret Mahoney, together
with Thomas W. Moloney and Robert Ebert, launched the Picker/
Commonwealth Program for Patient-Centered Care, and they have
been instrumental in shaping it. We also owe a particular debt of
gratitude to Robert Biblo, Mo Katz, and Amy Stursberg, our project
officers.

We rely throughout this volume on information gathered by
program staff and consultants and on the insights they have given
us. In this connection, we must first acknowledge Paul D. Cleary
of the Harvard Medical School, the program's director of research;
he has overseen the development of the survey instrument, its application in the field, and the analysis of its results. Humphrey
Taylor and Robert Leitman of Louis Harris and Associates also

participated in this work, and William McMullen of the Harvard Medical School assisted with the data analysis. Sheyman Seto Dunlap, Emily Fowler, and Carol Shepard conducted literature reviews and valuable background research during the program's earlier days. More recently, David Stokes has helped us analyze and understand our data and display them graphically, and Carolyn Slanetz helped us follow up information and check facts. Patricia Wilkinson has helped with our travel arrangements, provided secretarial support, and generally made our lives brighter.

Many consultants gave freely of their expertise, their powers of observation, and their time in helping us with our field visits to hospitals. We are grateful to Dennis Andrulis of the National Public Health and Hospital Institute; Laura Avakian of Boston's Beth Israel Hospital; James Bentley of the American Hospital Association; Richard Bogue of the Hospital Research and Educational Trust; David Bor of the Cambridge Hospital; Leonard Bushnell of Boston's Beth Israel Hospital; Daniel Couch of the Truman Medical Center in Kansas City, Missouri; Frank Davidoff of the American College of Physicians; David Dolins of Boston's Beth Israel Hospital; Trish Gibbons of Yale–New Haven Hospital; Thomas Gilmore of the Wharton Center for Applied Research; Barbara Giloth of the Hospital Research and Educational Trust; Nancy Kane and Christian Koeck from the Harvard School of Public Health; Seth Landefeld of Case Western Reserve University; Jane Lee of Methodist Hospitals, Houston; Mack Lipkin, Jr., of Bellevue Hospital; Maureen McCausland of Boston's Beth Israel Hospital; Ann Minnick of Rush–Presbyterian–St. Luke's Medical Center in Chicago; Ellen Powers of Boston's Beth Israel Hospital; Marilyn Sharpe of the UCLA Medical Center; and Roxane Spitzer-Lehman of St. Joseph Health System.

We would also like to thank, as a group, the administrators and staff at Clinton Memorial Hospital; Community Hospital at Glen Cove; Jackson–Madison County General Hospital; the Mayo Clinic, St. Marys Hospital, and Rochester Methodist Hospital; Medical College of Virginia Hospital; Mercy Medical Center; Newport Hospital; New York University Medical Center; California Pacific Medical Center and the Planetree Model Hospital Unit; the Regional Medical Center at Memphis; Riverside Methodist Hospital;

Salem Hospital; St. Elizabeth's Hospital Medical Center; St. Mary's Hospital and Medical Center; Trinity Medical Center; Tampa General Hospital; the University of Chicago Hospitals; and the University of Minnesota's Patient Learning Center.

The editors and contributing authors of this book are all associates of the Picker/Commonwealth Program for Patient-Centered Care—leaders, managers, and research investigators. Writing the book has been a collaborative effort. For the most part, we have arrived at the important editorial decisions through a process of consensus. And while each chapter is the unmistakable product of its author's creative thinking, each also bears the imprint of the long hours we spent together reviewing and criticizing drafts.

Boston, Massachusetts   Margaret Gerteis
March 1993   Susan Edgman-Levitan
                                                                               Jennifer Daley
                                                                               Thomas L. Delbanco

THE EDITORS

Margaret Gerteis is a staff associate in the Picker/Commonwealth Program for Patient-Centered Care. She received her B.A. degree (1968) from Antioch College in history and both her M.A. (1975) and Ph.D. (1985) degrees from Tufts University, also in history. In her professional life, Gerteis has pursued parallel interests in social history, organizational culture and behavior, and health policy. Prior to joining the Picker/Commonwealth Program in 1989, she conducted research on health and environmental policy for several years at the Harvard School of Public Health and served as deputy director of the school's Center for Health Communication from 1986 to 1989. She has coauthored scholarly articles appearing in the *Journal of Health Politics, Policy and Law, Health Affairs,* and other publications. She has also contributed to several books and written numerous case studies on issues relating to health and environmental policy.

Susan Edgman-Levitan is associate director and program manager of the Picker/Commonwealth Program. She received her B.A. degree (1973) from the University of Michigan in history and her P.A. (1977) magna cum laude from the Physician Assistant Program at Duke University. Edgman-Levitan's professional interests have focused on hospital- and community-based primary care, on strategies to enhance individuals' ability to live productively with illness, and on nontraditional approaches to healing. She worked for several years as a primary care physician's assistant in North Carolina and served as clinical associate professor at Duke University School of Medicine in Durham, North Carolina. Prior to joining the Picker/Commonwealth Program, Edgman-Levitan was director of planning at the Health and Hospitals Corporation of New York City. She is coeditor of *Medicine and Pediatrics* (1988, with J. D. Crapo and M. A. Hamilton), a textbook for medical students, physicians' assistants, and nurse practitioners.

Jennifer Daley is assistant professor of medicine at Harvard University, where she is a staff physician in the Division of General Medicine and Primary Care, Department of Medicine, Beth Israel Hospital, Boston. She is also a consultant to the Picker/Commonwealth Program, and a staff physician and associate director of Health Services Research and Primary Care at the Brockton/West Roxbury Veterans Affairs Medical Center, West Roxbury, Massachusetts. She received her B.A. degree (1972) from Brown University in human studies and her M.D. degree (1976) from Tufts University. She completed her internal medicine training at the New England Medical Center (1979) in Boston and completed a research fellowship (1987) in the General Medicine Faculty Development and Fellowship Program at Harvard Medical School. Daley's main research interests are in quality-of-care measurement, outcomes and effectiveness research, and risk adjustment methodologies. In addition to her numerous research publications, she is the author of the *Guidebook on Uses of Mortality Data: Applications in Hospital Quality Assurance Activities* (1990).

Thomas L. Delbanco is director of the Division of General Medicine and Primary Care at Boston's Beth Israel Hospital, associate professor of medicine at the Harvard Medical School, and director of the Picker/Commonwealth Program. He received his B.A. degree (1961) from Harvard College in government and his M.D. degree (1965) from Columbia College of Physicians and Surgeons. He trained in internal medicine at Bellevue, Harlem, and Presbyterian Hospitals in New York. Delbanco established one of the first primary care practices and teaching programs to be based in an academic health center. He has authored over a hundred scholarly papers and has coedited two books: *Alcoholism: A Guide for the Primary Care Physician* (1987, with H. B. Barnes and M. D. Aronson) and *Manual of Clinical Evaluation: Strategies for Cost-Effective Care* (1988, with M. D. Aronson). Delbanco is past president of the Society of General Internal Medicine and a member of the program committee of the Institute of Medicine, an organization of the National Academy of Sciences. In addition, he serves on the board of directors of the National Public Health and Hospitals Institute.

OTHER CONTRIBUTORS

Kimberly D. Allshouse is services coordinator for Howard County Services in Burlington, Vermont, and a consultant to the Picker/ Commonwealth Program for Patient-Centered Care. She received her B.A. degree (1983) from Dickinson College in philosophy and her M.S.W. degree (1990) from Boston University School of Social Work. Allshouse's professional work has been guided by her interest in ethics in health and social services. From 1988 to 1991, she served on the research staff of the Picker/Commonwealth Program, where she conducted background research on various aspects of patient-centered care and helped organize the program's national survey of hospital patients. Allshouse is a contributing author to several scholarly articles and the coauthor of a forthcoming working paper, "Resiliency Amidst Inequity: Older Women Workers in an Aging United States" (with P. Rayman).

Beth Ellers is a research consultant to the Picker/Commonwealth Program for Patient-Centered Care. She received her B.A. degree (1975) from Bryn Mawr College in anthropology, her M.D. degree (1984) from the Medical College of Pennsylvania, and her M.P.H. degree (1988) from the Harvard School of Public Health. Ellers also trained in pediatrics at Brown University's Rhode Island Hospital, and her primary professional interests are in maternal and child health and childhood injury prevention. In addition to her work with the Picker/Commonwealth Program, she chairs the Prevention of Poverty Study Group of the Coalition for Maine's Children and is active in childhood advocacy projects in her home state of Maine.

Thomas W. Moloney is director of Public Policy and Health Care Programs at the Institute for the Future. He received his B.A. degree (1967) from Colgate University in mathematics and philosophy. He received his M.A. degree (1970) in education, his M.P.H. degree (1971) in hospital administration, and his M.B.A. degree (1973) in finance and accounting, all from Columbia University. From 1980 to 1992, Moloney was senior vice president of The Commonwealth Fund of New York, where he had primary responsibility for conceptualizing, developing, and managing domestic programs that aimed to improve the caliber of individuals' lives and their opportunities for growing up, growing older, and staying healthy. He is the author of numerous articles in such journals as *Health Affairs, New England Journal of Medicine,* and the *Journal of the American Medical Association.* He is also coeditor of *New Approaches to the Medicaid Crisis* (1982, with R. J. Blendon).

Barbara Paul is director of policy analysis at Montefiore Medical Center, Bronx, New York. She received her B.A. degree (1975) from Carleton College in English and her M.A. degree (1982) from the University of Minnesota in journalism. From 1986 to 1992, she was a member of the program staff of The Commonwealth Fund of New York, where she worked closely with the Picker/Commonwealth Program. Paul's work focuses on examining and seeking ways to reconcile the differing perspectives, interests, and pursuits of the various participant groups in the American health care system. She is the author of numerous reports and monographs on aspects of health care. Articles she has coauthored with Thomas W. Moloney have appeared in *Health Affairs.*

Marc J. Roberts is professor of political economy and health policy and a member of the faculty at both the Harvard School of Public Health and the John F. Kennedy School of Government, as well as being a consultant to the Picker/Commonwealth Program. He received both his B.A. (1964) and his Ph.D. (1969) degrees from Harvard in economics. Roberts has studied and written widely on public policy problems, with a focus on environmental regulation and the organization of health care services. His more recent publications include *The Search for Safety: Chemicals and Cancer Risk* (1988, with J. D. Graham and L. C. Green) and *The Environmental Protection Agency: Asking the Wrong Questions* (1990, with M. K. Landy and S. R. Thomas). From 1987 to 1991, he was associate director of the Picker/Commonwealth Program. A former chair of the Department of Health Policy and Management at the Harvard School of Public Health, Roberts now serves as faculty chair of the Kennedy School's Executive Program for Senior Managers in State and Local Government and of the Senior Executive Fellows Program for career federal civil servants.

Janice D. Walker is assistant director of the Picker/Commonwealth Program. She received her B.S.N. degree (1977) from the University of Kansas and her M.B.A. degree (1984) from Boston University School of Management. Walker's professional work has focused on the development of systems to evaluate the cost and quality of care. She was previously a senior consultant at the Health Data Institute (a subsidiary of Baxter Healthcare Corporation), where she directed a variety of projects for government and private sector clients involving clinical audits, insurance benefits modeling, and commercial software development. Walker is a former staff nurse at Boston City Hospital and former head nurse in its coronary care and progressive care units. She has coauthored several scholarly papers on quality-of-care data and related topics of health care management and finance. Her articles, coauthored, have appeared in the *Journal of the American Medical Association*.

Through the Patient's Eyes

INTRODUCTION:
Medicine and Health
from the Patient's Perspective

Margaret Gerteis
Susan Edgman-Levitan
Jennifer Daley
Thomas L. Delbanco

Some years ago, when officials in Massachusetts tried to close a small and foundering community hospital in the north-central part of the state, busloads of loyal patients and angry citizens descended on the State House in protest and ultimately fought the effort all the way to the Supreme Judicial Court of the Commonwealth. Health planners were bewildered. The decision to close Winchendon Hospital was based on an objective assessment of areawide needs and available resources; it was part of a plan to create a more rational, efficient, and less costly statewide health system. There were good and well-known reasons for closing the hospital: it had fewer than fifty beds; it had an outdated physical plant in serious violation of health, fire, and safety codes; and it was unequipped to handle even the most routine inpatient care. Most of the doctors who treated Winchendon's patients already had admitting privileges at one of two larger, newer, well-equipped, and underutilized hospitals within a fifteen- or twenty-minute drive of the town center. And most patients were already accustomed to going either to these institutions or to the internationally renowned academic health centers in Boston to be treated for serious ailments (Gerteis, 1980).

Why, then, the hue and cry? The loyalty to Winchendon Hospital was partly an expression of community pride, but it was also deeper and more personal. Even though circumstances often dictated treatment elsewhere, townspeople preferred to be sick in their own hospital. There, you were among friends and neighbors who most likely knew you, your family, and your situation in life without having to be told. The care they gave you was personal, kindly, attentive. It was comforting. The same could *not* be said of every hospital, however sophisticated its diagnostic and therapeutic armamentaria. One woman, writing in defense of Winchendon Hospital, compared it favorably to one of the most prestigious medical institutions in Boston: "I had occasion to be at your Mass. General Hospital when my brother was operated on," she wrote in a letter to the governor. "As to the care he got—well, I would put our facility up against yours anytime. No bath or back rub for a week and a room that looked like a prison cell. Our cheery little hospital would put Mass. General to shame" (Gerteis, 1980, part A, p. 9). It was a theme that was repeated again and again during the months and years of battles over Winchendon's fate.

Winchendon Hospital ultimately closed, in spite of the zeal and legal victories of its defenders. The central planners had been right, in many ways: the hospital could not provide the quality of medical care demanded in the 1980s. The forces mitigating against smallness and insularity were too strong. Even the loyal patients of Winchendon knew that, as their pattern of admissions to other hospitals showed. They understood the necessity of being cared for by strangers when they were really sick (Rosenberg, 1987). Still, the outburst over the hospital's closure revealed a fatal weakness in the strategies of the health planners: objective, rational plans failed to take into account the subjective experience of patients. And patients' behavior never quite conformed to the planners' designs.

Science, Medicine, and the Quality of Experience

Quality in health and medical care, as the Winchendon story suggests, has two dimensions: one is objective, technical; the other is subjective and qualitative. However dazzling the technological achievements of medical science over the last fifty years, the patient's experience of illness and medical care is at the heart of the first purpose of clinical medicine—to relieve human suffering. Suffering, as practicing clinicians know, is a subjective experience that may or may not respond to therapeutic regimens directed toward the pathological processes of disease, even when those regimens are technically effective (Cassell, 1982; Kleinman, Eisenberg, and Good, 1978; Baron, 1985). Clinicians also know the dilemmas that arise when the "cure" feels worse than the disease, and the effect such contradictions have on clinical decision making, treatment efficacy, and clinical outcomes (Forrow, Wartman, and Brock, 1988; Brody, 1980; Kassirer and Pauker, 1981; Scheff, 1963; Feinstein, 1983a). From the early years of this century, when eminent physicians like Richard Cabot at the Massachusetts General Hospital struggled with the incongruities of Christian compassion and scientific distance, to modern times, when the proponents of clinical decision analysis struggle with the cerebral task of quantifying individual values, medical practitioners have searched for ways to reconcile the unique, subjective, and qualitative characteristics of sickness with the rationalist, objective, and categorical demands of medical science (Forrow, Wartman, and Brock, 1988; Kassirer and Pauker, 1981; Feinstein, 1983a, 1983b; Kassirer, Moskowitz, Lau, and Pauker, 1987; Read and others, 1984).

What patients experience, and what they think of that experience, should also matter to health care planners, policy makers, and managers, because that experience, as much as the technical quality of care, will determine how people use the health care system and how they benefit from it. Do patients get what they need from the facilities and services we design and manage? They expect, as a matter of course, that the care they receive will be technically sophisticated and up to date, although these may not be qualities they can readily judge. Their choices and decisions will largely be based on other factors. The interest demonstrated in recent years in measuring patient satisfaction, as well as its effect on choices of providers and medical plan enrollment patterns, is testimony to the magnitude of concern among planners and third-party payers to understand why patients make the choices they do (Dimatteo, Taranta, Friedman, and Prince, 1980; Weiss and Senf, 1990; Pope, 1978; Linn and others, 1985; Davies and others, 1986; Murray, 1987; Marquis, Davies, and Ware, 1983; Ware and Davies, 1983). So, too, the number of management tools and consultative services now available—from patient-satisfaction surveys and modest "guest relations" programs to long-range strategies for total customer-driven quality improvement—attests to managers' recognition of the competitive implications of patients' perceptions (Press, Ganey, and Malone, 1991; Omachonu, 1990; Steiber, 1988).

For the most part, those who work in the health care field do not need to be convinced that what patients think, feel, and experience is important. Health professionals are, by nature, a kind and sensitive lot, motivated by an honest desire to help people and ease their suffering. But if they recognize the intrinsic importance of patients' subjective experience to the quality of care, why has that experience not figured more prominently in shaping health care services and institutions? Why has there not been a more systematic effort to incorporate patients' experiences and judgments into planning and quality assessment? In part, the answer lies with the fundamental tension between the objectively analytical tendencies of medicine as science and the subjective and personal nature of medicine as practice. The ideology of science, which has shaped medical training for most of this century, values that which is quantifiable, generalizable, and amenable to technical intervention. The qualitative, individual, and human aspects of the patient's experience are hard to describe or evaluate in a way that is accepted as scientifically valid, even when they are acknowledged to be important (Forrow, Wartman, and Brock, 1988; Baron, 1985; Feinstein, 1983a; Entralgo, 1969). The practical difficulties that clinical decision analysts have encountered in their attempts to quantify individual utilities reflect this dilemma (Kassirer, Moskowitz, Lau, and Pauker, 1987), as we will see in Chapter Two.

The institutional setting of health care in the late twentieth century, however critical it may be to the delivery of high-quality and high-tech medical care, also tends, by its very nature, to depersonalize the clinical encounter. It removes patients from their natural social environment of home, family, and community; sorts them into diagnostic or functional groupings defined by the institution and its professional staff; and treats them using processes, protocols, and procedures deemed appropriate to each category (Entralgo, 1969). The institutionalization or rational organization of health services need not by itself compromise the quality of patient-centered care. But health care institutions are complex organizations that have developed to serve many constituents besides patients. And their work has come to be both defined and limited by the systems and structures that have evolved to carry out competing functions. As our colleagues in the quality consulting business remind us, problems lie not with people, but with systems.

Defining a Conceptual Framework: The Dimensions of Patient-Centered Care

Our focus in the chapters that follow is on the patient's experience of illness and health care and the systems that work, and fail to work, to meet patients' needs, as they define them. We use the term *patient-centered care* to describe an approach that consciously adopts the patient's perspective. What is it about their interaction with providers, systems, and institutions that patients say matters to them and affects them, either positively or negatively? To answer this question, we first convened three focus groups of recently discharged medical and surgical patients and their family members from the Boston area and asked them to talk about their hospital experiences. To make sure that our sample of Boston-area patients did not have a perspective markedly different from that of patients elsewhere in the country, we developed a brief questionnaire based on the focus-group discussions and conducted open-ended telephone interviews with fifty patients from five hospitals across the country, along with fifty of their family members or friends. Using focus groups of physicians and non-physician hospital staff and a review of the pertinent literature to help flesh out the context of the patients' observations, we then defined seven primary dimensions of patient-centered care, as outlined below.

1. Respect for Patients' Values, Preferences, and Expressed Needs

Focus group patients described a sense of anonymity and loss of identity in the hospital and a strong need to be recognized and treated with dignity and respect as individuals. They also worried about how their sickness or treatment might affect their lives, and they wanted to be both informed about and involved in the medical decisions that might affect their lives. Respecting patients' individuality and restoring their autonomy entails paying attention to the following:

Quality of Life. What impact does the illness or treatment have on the patients' quality of life or subjective sense of well-being? How is this mediated by life-style, cultural values, or religious beliefs? How can health care help patients achieve their short-term and long-term goals? What are the limitations of treatment?

Involvement in Decision Making. What level of involvement do patients want in decision making? How does this vary over time, or with the degree of illness? How much, and to whom (clinician, family, friends), would patients prefer to defer to others?

Dignity. Are patients' physical and emotional needs for privacy and individual expression respected? Are they treated with dignity, respect, and sensitivity to their cultural values? Do staff treat patients kindly and respectfully?

Needs and Autonomy. What do patients need, want, or expect from their encounter with a health care provider or system? How do these needs and expectations differ from those perceived by providers? How much can patients do on their own, and how much do they want to do? How does this mesh with the provider's demands or expectations?

2. Coordination and Integration of Care

Patients in focus groups expressed a strong feeling of vulnerability and powerlessness in the face of illness, and the need for competent and caring medical staff that could inspire their immediate and unqualified trust. Their perceptions of the competence and efficiency of their caregivers are shaped, in large part, by three distinct tasks of coordination, unique to the environment of hospitals and health care facilities:

Coordination and Integration of Clinical Care. Who is in charge of the patient's care? Is that person recognized by the patient, as well as by the members of the clinical team? How are clinical services coordinated? Do members of the team communicate effectively among each other and deliver a consistent set of messages to the patient and family?

Coordination and Integration of Ancillary and Support Services. Are the needs and perceptions of patients, as well as of clinicians, taken into account? Are jobs defined in terms of patient care as well as technical function? Do components of ancillary systems work together smoothly and effectively, and does information go to the right person at the right time? Do patients and their families understand what services, procedures, or consultations are to be ordered, when they are to occur, what they will require of the patients, and how patients might be affected?

Coordination and Integration of "Front-Line" Patient Care. Does the patient know whom to ask for help? Is the right person available at the right time? Is front-line staff knowledgeable about the patient, and do they have the information they need to do their job? Do staff have the administrative and organizational support they need to deliver patient care? Are direct patient care functions that cross bureaucratic lines effectively coordinated?

3. Information, Communication, and Education

Patients often express the fear that information is being withheld from them, that they are not being completely or honestly informed about their illness or prognosis. In particular, focus group patients and providers emphasized the need for the following:

Information on Clinical Status, Progress, and Prognosis. Do patients get the information they want about their clinical status, progress, or prognosis? Is it delivered in language that they can understand? Is it consistently kept up to date? Are patients and their families informed of major changes in a timely way?

Information on Processes of Care. Are test results explained to patients and their families in language they can understand? Do they understand how alternative treatment regimens might affect their subjective well-being as well as their clinical status? Do they understand the reasoning behind clinical decisions?

Information and Education to Facilitate Autonomy, Self-Care, and Health Promotion. Do patients and their families know what they need to know to manage on their own, to the extent that they desire and are able to do so? Do they understand how they can help (or hinder) recovery and prevent illness in the future?

4. Physical Comfort

One of the most immediately disturbing aspects of illness is the physical discomfort and disability it brings. Physical care that comforts patients, especially when they are acutely ill, is therefore one of the most elemental services that caregivers can provide, from the patients' perspective. Focus group patients also reported a heightened awareness of the cold, frightening, or gloomy institutional trappings of the hospital environment, and a parallel appreciation of clean, comfortable, and pleasant surroundings. The most basic components of physical comfort include the following:

Pain Management. Do staff listen to patients' complaints about pain or requests for pain medication and respond in a timely and effective way? Are patients and their families told how much pain to expect as a result of illness, tests, or procedures? Do staff explain to them how their pain can be managed? Is their pain alleviated as much as possible?

Help with Activities of Daily Living. Are patients given the help they need with using the toilet, bathing, grooming, eating, and so forth? Are their needs for privacy and cultural values accommodated?

Surroundings and Hospital Environment. Are patient areas kept clean, comfortable, and reasonably pleasant? Are they accessible to friends and family and easy to find? Is equipment that may provoke fear or anxiety kept out of sight as much as possible? Are patients' needs for privacy accommodated?

5. *Emotional Support and Alleviation of Fear and Anxiety*

The fears and anxieties that illness provokes may be as debilitating as the physical effects. In particular, caregivers need to pay attention to the following:

Anxiety Over Clinical Status, Treatment, and Prognosis. Are patients anxious about their illness, worried about treatment, fearful of the outcome or prognosis? What are those fears? Do patients have a relationship of confidence and trust with staff members who can address their fears? Are those people accessible? Do the staff members have the information needed to answer the patients' questions? Is it communicated effectively? Is the information conveyed in a way that alleviates, rather than exacerbates, fear?

Anxiety Over the Impact of the Illness on Self and Family. Are patients worried about the impact of the illness on their ability to care for themselves or dependents? Are there people on staff who can help with those concerns or provide appropriate referrals? Are those people knowledgeable and accessible? What emotional impact does the illness have on patients' friends and family? Are supports available to them?

Anxiety over the Financial Impact of the Illness. Are patients concerned about paying for their medical care or hospitalization? Are there staff who can help with those concerns or make appropriate referrals? Are patients worried about losing income as a result of disability? Are there staff members who can help with those worries?

6. *Involvement of Family and Friends*

The central role of family members and close friends in patients' experience of illness was a continuing theme of the patient focus groups. At the same time, patients worried about the repercussions their illness would have on friends and family members. The family dimension of patient-centered care entails the following:

Accommodation of Family and Friends. Who do patients rely on for social and emotional support? Are they recognized and accommodated by clinicians and caregivers? What impact might they have on the patients' clinical course or subjective experience of illness? To what extent do the patients view the involvement of some friends or family members in negative terms?

Involving Family in Decision Making. Do patients look to family or friends to act as advocate, proxy, or surrogate? Are those people's roles recognized and respected by hospital staff? Do they have the information needed to play their roles effectively? Alternatively, do patients prefer to withhold information from friends and family? Are those preferences respected?

Supporting the Family as Caregiver. Are family or friends able to provide physical support and care for the patients on an immediate or extended basis? Are they encouraged and supported in that role? Do they have the information and skills they need to be effective?

Recognizing the Needs of the Family. What impacts does the illness have on family dynamics and functioning? What effect might this have on the patients' clinical course or subjective well-being? What forms of support and assistance do they need, and what resources are available to help them?

7. *Transition and Continuity*

Focus group patients expressed considerable anxiety about their ability to care for themselves away from the clinical setting. Attending to this dimension of patient-centered care entails taking the following into account:

Information. Do patients and family understand medications to take, dietary or treatment regimens to follow, and danger signals to look out for after leaving the hospital or health care facility? Do patients and family know what to do to help or hinder recovery, promote health, or prevent the recurrence of disease?

Coordination and Planning. Have plans been made and services coordinated to ensure continuing care and treatment? Do patients and/or family understand these plans?

Support. Do patients and family have access to clinical, social, physical, and financial supports on a continuing basis? Do they understand how to get that support and whom to call for help?

Assessing the Status of Patient-Centered Care: Quantitative and Qualitative Data

With this framework in mind, we set out to explore the status of patient-centered care in the United States. Our first task was to develop a survey instrument that would elicit specific reports from patients about the aspects of care they perceived as important, in lieu of the satisfaction ratings generally used on patient surveys (Cleary and others, 1991). Based on the focus-group findings, we developed a list of statements reflecting specific experiences or aspects of care patients had mentioned—for example, "After surgery, the anesthesiologist came to see how the patient was doing," or "The nurse asked the patient about his worries." We then asked groups of physicians, nurses, and health experts familiar with the patient's perspective to review the statements and assess their importance. Items that were not considered important to any of the three groups were dropped, unless the patient focus groups had deemed them especially important. The remaining statements were then turned into sixty-two interview questions. For the purposes of analysis, we also included questions about respondents' social and demographic characteristics, length of stay, the nature of their hospital admission, health status, and disability days. Two broadly similar but distinct interview protocols were developed: one for use with patients and one for use with friends or family members ("care partners") closely involved in their hospital care. The interview was pilot-tested (in English and Spanish) with a sample of about 400 patients recently discharged from fourteen hospitals in different parts of the country.

Using the 1988 American Hospital Association Hospital Survey data base, we then selected a stratified probability sample of hospitals in the continental United States. All eligible hospitals (general acute care nonfederal and nonprofit hospitals with more than 100 beds) were stratified by ownership (public or private nonprofit), geographical location (East, South, Midwest, or West), and teaching status (academic health centers, other teaching hospitals, or nonteaching hospitals). Sixty-two hospitals agreed to participate in the study. Each participating hospital provided us with a list of all adult medical and surgical patients discharged during the preceding month. From this, we selected a random sample of approximately 100 eligible patients from each hospital to be interviewed within six months after their discharge. Louis Harris and Associates, Inc., conducted interviews by telephone between March 1, 1989 and November 5, 1989, with a total of 6,455 selected patients and approximately 2,000 of their identified care partners. Interviews were conducted in English and Spanish.

Our purpose in conducting the survey was threefold. First, we wanted to assess the status of patient-centered care in the country, to determine, if we could, what substance lies beneath the widespread stories of disenchantment with the health care system. Second, we wished to know whether some patients were more "at risk" than others—for example, those who were poorer, older, sicker, or without medical insurance. And finally, we wanted to know how much the quality of patient-centered care varied from one hospital to another, and in what patterns. We have reported the major findings from the survey in some detail elsewhere (Cleary and others, 1991). The survey helped us find hospitals in our sample that were doing better at providing patient-centered care than others, but it could not tell us why they were doing better or how they were doing it. To help answer these questions, we organized interdisciplinary teams of clinicians, hospital administrators, social scientists, and others, including members of the program staff as well as outside consultants, to visit selected sites. Among these were hospitals and programs that had come to our attention for particular innovations in patient-centered care, as well as those we selected on the basis of their performance on our national survey. In all, we visited twenty different sites. Our aim in these one-day visits was to explore in a general way management practices and organizational characteristics affecting patient-centered care and to learn more about the design and operation of particular programs.

The following chapters are based on the information thus gathered for this project from focus groups, the national survey, site visits, and reviews of the literature. Our purpose is to share what we have learned and to suggest a structured way to think about the quality of health care from the patient's perspective and incorporate that perspective into quality assessment. We aim to point out not only the barriers in current systems of health care, but also the practical opportunities for improvement. Our focus, given the particular history of this project, is primarily on hospitals. But as the locus of care shifts more and more to outpatient settings, our findings and observations will become increasingly relevant to ambulatory clinics and physicians' offices as well. We have framed the discussion with these larger interests in mind.

References

Baron, R. J. "An Introduction to Medical Phenomenology: I Can't Hear You While I'm Listening." *Annals of Internal Medicine,* 1985, *103,* 606–611.

Brody, D. S. "The Patient's Role in Clinical Decision-Making." *Annals of Internal Medicine,* 1980, *93,* 718–722.

Cassell, E. J. "The Nature of Suffering and the Goals of Medicine." *New England Journal of Medicine,* 1982, *306,* 639–645.

Cleary, P. D., and others. "Patients Evaluate Their Hospital Care: A National Survey." *Health Affairs,* 1991, *10,* 254–267.

Davies, A. R., and others. "Consumer Acceptance of Prepaid and Fee-for-Service Medical Care: Results from a Randomized Controlled Trial." *Health Services Research,* 1986, *21,* 429.

Dimatteo, M. R., Taranta, A., Friedman, H. S., and Prince, L. M. "Predicting Patient Satisfaction from Physicians' Nonverbal Communication Skills." *Medical Care,* 1980, *18,* 376–387.

Entralgo, P. L. *Doctor and Patient.* New York: McGraw-Hill, 1969.

Feinstein, A. R. "An Additional Basic Science for Clinical Medicine. 1: The Constraining Fundamental Paradigms." *Annals of Internal Medicine,* 1983a, *99,* 393–397.

Feinstein, A. R. "An Additional Basic Science for Clinical Medicine. 2: The Limitations of Randomized Trials." *Annals of Internal Medicine,* 1983b, *99,* 544–550.

Forrow, L., Wartman, S. A., and Brock, D. W. "Science, Ethics, and the Making of Clinical Decisions: Implications for Risk Factor Intervention." *Journal of the American Medical Association,* 1988, *259,* 3161–3167.

Gerteis, M. "Winchendon Hospital." Case study, parts A, B, C. Curriculum Resource Center, Harvard School of Public Health, 1980.

Kassirer, J. P., and Pauker, S. G. "The Toss-Up." *New England Journal of Medicine,* 1981, *305,* 1467–1469.

Kassirer, J. P., Moskowitz, A. J., Lau, J., and Pauker, S. G. "Decision Analysis: A Progress Report." *Annals of Internal Medicine,* 1987, *106,* 275–291.

Kleinman, A., Eisenberg, L., and Good, B. "Culture, Illness, and Care: Clinical Lessons from Anthropologic and Cross-Cultural Research." *Annals of Internal Medicine,* 1978, *88,* 251–258.

Linn, L. S., and others. "Physician and Patient Satisfaction as Factors Related to the Organization of Internal Medicine Group Practices." *Medical Care,* 1985, *23,* 1171–1178.

Marquis, M. S., Davies, A. R., and Ware, J. E. "Patient Satisfaction and Change in Medical Care Provider: A Longitudinal Study." *Medical Care,* 1983, *21,* 821.

Murray, J. P. "A Comparison of Patient Satisfaction Among Prepaid and Fee-for-Service Patients." *Journal of Family Practice,* 1987, *24,* 203–207.

Omachonu, V. K. "Quality of Care and the Patient: New Criteria for Evaluation." *Health Care Management Review,* 1990, *15,* 43–50.

Pope, C. R. "Consumer Satisfaction in a Health Maintenance Organization." *Journal of Health and Social Behavior,* 1978, *19,* 291–303.

Press, I., Ganey, R. F., and Malone, M. P. "Satisfied Patients Can Spell Financial Well-Being." *Healthcare Financial Management,* 1991, *45*(2), 34–40.

Read, J. L., and others. "Preferences for Health Outcomes: Comparison of Assessment Methods." *Medical Decision Making,* 1984, *4,* 315–329.

Rosenberg, C. E. *The Care of Strangers: The Rise of America's Hospital System.* New York: Basic Books, 1987.

Scheff, T. J. "Decision Rules, Types of Error, and Their Consequences in Medical Diagnosis." *Behavioral Science,* 1963, *8,* 97–107.

Steiber, S. R. "How Consumers Perceive Health Care Quality." *Hospitals,* Apr. 5, 1988, p. 84.

Ware, J. E., Jr., and Davies, A. R. "Behavioral Consequences of Consumer Dissatisfaction with Medical Care." *Evaluation and Program Planning,* 1983, *6,* 291.

Weiss, B. D., and Senf, J. H. "Patient Satisfaction Survey Instrument for Use in Health Maintenance Organizations." *Medical Care,* 1990, *28,* 434–445.

PART I

The Dimensions
of Patient-Centered Care

2

Treating
Patients as Individuals

Kimberly D. Allshouse

Patients are usually satisfied with the technical quality of care they receive. But somewhere in the process, their individuality is lost sight of; their personal and subjective needs remain unmet. "I felt I was grist for the mill," one focus group patient observed, "just pushing along at a routine rate, just another appendix . . . or another tumor lying on the table." Too often, the technology drives the system. Time is limited. Taking a few minutes to listen to patients' concerns, questions, needs, and goals may be neither encouraged nor rewarded. Health care providers often recognize the paradox that comes with reliance on technology. One physician's inadvertent slip of the tongue captured the essence of the problem: "It happened the other morning on rounds, as it often does, that while I was carefully auscultating a patient's chest, he began to ask me a question. 'Quiet,' I said, 'I can't hear you while I'm listening'" (Baron, 1985, p. 606).

And yet the system faces challenges on several fronts. Perhaps most noticeably, patients themselves, as they become more knowledgeable consumers of health care, demand change. As high-technology medical care dramatically expands treatment options, it also raises unprecedented moral and ethical questions that clinicians are unequipped to answer alone. And the growing cultural diversity of our nation makes it increasingly difficult, even hazardous, to overlook the heterogeneity among patients and the idiosyncrasies that have always been there.

19

Respecting patients' individuality is the foundation of humane medical care. It requires confronting the fullness of the human context in which illness occurs. A theme that will resound throughout this book, whether we are discussing ways to educate patients, how to meet their emotional needs, or the role of family and friends, is that individual patients must be the focus of attention, that their particular concerns must be recognized and addressed. Here, we focus on the broad aspects of respecting patients' individuality: understanding how cultural beliefs, values, and practices affect their perceptions of illness and expectations for treatment; eliciting and respecting their preferences for involvement in clinical care; and elucidating patients' therapeutic goals and weighing appropriate treatment options.

Understanding and Respecting
Cultural Beliefs and Practices

"I've heard of people with snakes in their body. . . . And they take 'em someplace to a witch doctor and snakes come out. My sister . . . had . . . a snake that was in her arm. . . . This thing was just runnin' up her arm, whatever it was, just runnin' up her arm. . . . You could actually see it when she would go into one of her spells, it was in her left arm. Some woman they said didn't like her [had put it there]" (quoted in Snow, 1974, p. 86). Descriptions like this one, given by an elderly black American from the rural South, illustrate dramatically how discordant a patient's explanation of illness can be with the scientific, medical explanatory model that guides most clinical practice. Health care providers who routinely treat new immigrants from Latin America, Southeast Asia, Arab countries, the Caribbean, or Eastern Europe confront equally exotic health beliefs and practices that complicate the task of diagnosis, treatment, communication, and care. And yet all patients, regardless of their ethnicity or degree of socialization, bring culturally defined beliefs and practices to the experience of illness that shape their encounters with the health care system and their response to clinical care. Here, we examine the importance of culture in both patients' and clinicians' explanatory models of health and disease and their impact on health-related behavior. And finally, we suggest how these beliefs can be elicited and incorporated into plans of patient care.

Illness Versus Disease

A large part of the cultural discord that exists between patients and clinicians lies in the inherent difference between the patients' subjective experience of "illness" and the clinician's objective approach to "disease" (Baron, 1981, 1985; Cassell, 1982, 1984; Eisenberg, 1977; Hautman, 1979; Helman, 1990; Kleinman, Eisenberg, and Good, 1978; Spector, 1979). To a patient, illness entails not only the physical discomfort of ill health, but all of the social and psychological ramifications of being unwell. And the broader meaning of illness in this emotional and social context—its effect on their lives and on the lives of those around them—may be far more important to patients than the physical impairment itself (Helman, 1990; Kleinman, Eisenberg, and Good, 1978). It is the experience of illness that patients bring to the health care system. As Baron (1981, p. 21) observes, "People do not come in for diagnosis and treatment; they come to be made well, made whole, to recover the sense of health, of being well, fully alive, in-the-world."

But if illness is, in Cassell's (1976, p. 27) words, "what the patient feels when he goes to the doctor," then disease is "what he has on the way home from the doctor's office." It is disease, not illness, that health care providers are equipped to treat. In the clinician's eyes, as Baron observes (1981, p. 7), "the patient comes to function as a kind of translucent screen on which the disease is projected." Carried to its extreme, the biomedical focus of medicine can result in what Kleinman, Eisenberg, and Good (1978, p. 252) have called "a veterinary practice of medicine." The experience of illness becomes irrelevant, except as it reveals the underlying presence of disease. The patient's sociocultural identity—the sum of the person's beliefs, practices, habits, norms, customs, and rituals—only clouds the screen. Modern medicine has been described, with only a hint of jest, as so disease oriented that the ideal situation would be to have patients leave their damaged physical vessels at the hospital for repair, while taking their social and emotional selves home (Lorber, 1975).

And yet for many patients, the problems of illness—the difficulties in daily living that result from ill-health—constitute the entire disorder. It is from illness in this sense that they seek relief. As one physician we interviewed acknowledged, "patients don't necessarily experience their needs as, 'I need to have a diagnosis made,' and 'I need to have treatment.'" If health care institutions are to meet patients' needs, they need to understand and confront patients' experience of illness within this larger cultural context.

Explanatory Models of Illness

The cause of ill-health in many folk medical traditions is often supernatural, metaphysical, or interpersonal. In traditional Hispanic cultures, the source of sickness could be a "hot" and "cold" imbalance, or the dislocation of internal organs, or it may have a magical or emotional origin (Hautman, 1979). Hispanic patients may speak of *susto*, an illness arising from fright, or *empacho*, stomach cramps believed to be caused by a ball of food sticking to the wall of the stomach (Spector, 1979). Chinese patients may believe that illness is caused by an imbalance of *yin* and *yang*. Many Native Americans feel that the source of sickness lies in a lack of harmony or an imbalance with natural or supernatural forces (Hautman, 1979). Black Americans from the rural South may believe that sickness is a divine punishment for sin or a sign of disharmony with the forces of nature (Snow, 1974).

Patients and clinicians bring their own explanatory models to an episode of illness, shaped by culture, education, and experience (Kleinman, Eisenberg, and Good, 1978). These preexisting beliefs form their understanding of the etiology of the illness, its symptoms, the pathophysiological processes involved, the likely course and the seriousness of the illness, and the appropriate treatments. The discrepancy between patients' and clinicians' understanding of illness may be particularly striking when they come from very different social and cultural backgrounds (Helman, 1990). From a biomedical perspective, such folk explanations of ill-health as *susto* or *empacho* may be dismissed as scientifically unfounded. And patients whose health beliefs deviate markedly from the biomedical model may therefore be reluctant to discuss their practices and beliefs, for fear of ridicule (Berlin and Fowkes, 1983). And yet even patients from social and educational backgrounds broadly similar to those of their caregivers often have different explanatory models that affect their understanding of illness and their behavior. Kleinman, Eisenberg, and Good (1978) cite the case of a thirty-eight-year old university professor, for example, who insisted that he be diagnosed as having a pulmonary embolus, instead of angina pectoris, because (as it turned out) angina in his mind signaled the onset of semi-invalidism. Another case involved a white Protestant plumber's wife, whose understanding of her own "plumbing" caused her to purge herself relentlessly in an effort to get rid of what had been described to her as "water in the lungs."

Unless caregivers understand how *patients* understand their illness and discuss those beliefs with them, the effectiveness of any treatment may be seriously compromised. Underlying disagreements about the source of ill-health or the appropriate treatment can lead to medicolegal problems, problems with clinical management, poor compliance, and poor care. The university professor in the case cited above angrily accused his cardiologist of misdiagnosis. The bizarre behavior of the plumber's wife baffled her caregivers. A Guatemalan woman being treated for severe regional enteritis with intravenous hyperalimentation and a restriction of all oral intake believed her doctors had written her off, because she could no longer eat and maintain a balance of "hot" and "cold" nutrients. She became angry, withdrawn, and uncooperative (Kleinman, Eisenberg, and Good, 1978).

The successful clinical relationship, as Helman (1990) points out, is one where patient and caregiver arrive at a consensus concerning etiology, diagnostic labels, physiological processes, prognosis, and optimal treatment. In each of the cases cited above, such a consensus was eventually reached, once the underlying explanatory models were understood (Kleinman, Eisenberg, and Good, 1978).

Culturally-Rooted Behaviors and Practices

Culture shapes not only what patients and clinicians believe about health and illness, but how they act in clinical situations and how they expect others to act. Virtually all of the conventions of everyday life, as well as those relating to illness in particular, are defined by culture, and the success of any social encounter depends on a common, or compatible, understanding of these conventions. They include all the unspoken norms that govern forms of address, attitudes toward authority, directness of speech, and displays of emotion; the norms that delineate "personal space" and define hygienic and dietary practices, as well as taboos about nudity and sexuality; and the norms that define gender, social, and family roles and the rituals pertaining to sickness and death.

Zola (1966) observed that culturally defined norms governing patterns of speech and appropriate displays of emotion affect the way patients communicate about their health problems and present symptoms and how clinicians respond. Italian-Americans, he found, tended to present their illness in a more voluble, emotional, and dramatic way than Irish-Americans. They also complained of more symptoms and stressed their negative impact. The Irish-Americans in his study, by contrast, tended to minimize their symptoms. This "language of distress" (Helman, 1990) also influenced physicians' choice of a diagnostic label. When no organic cause of complaint was found, the Italian-American patients in Zola's study were often labeled "neurotic" or otherwise psychologically disordered, while the Irish-Americans were given a nondiagnosis, such as "nothing found on tests." In a professional, medical culture that highly regards emotional control, the behavior of the Italian-Americans was apparently found deviant enough to warrant its own diagnostic designation (Zola, 1966).

Misunderstandings about culturally sanctioned customs and behavior are also prevalent. Some Native Americans burn sage during purification rituals, for example, but they may be accused of smoking marijuana when they do this in a hospital setting. In Western society, eye contact indicates sincere interest or understanding, but in other cultures, it may show disrespect. Compared to those from Eastern cultures, Westerners tend to interpret gender roles liberally; health care practitioners should not be surprised to find an African or Asian man refusing to be examined by a female doctor, or an African or Asian woman expecting her husband to be present throughout a consultation (Qureshi, 1989). In many Far

Eastern cultures, it is inappropriate for a female patient to discuss "female problems" in the presence of a male stranger—and this may pose particular problems of communication when a male interpreter is used. Russian immigrants may feel that handshaking and smiling signify frivolity and immaturity, and they may therefore have no confidence in a clinician who displays such behavior (Rothenburger, 1990). In Eastern cultures, rectal examinations and therapeutic agents (enemas, suppositories) are all taboo, and a psychiatric referral may make a person ineligible for an arranged marriage (Qureshi, 1989). Patients from cultures in which extended family members routinely gather around the sick may also run up against hospital restrictions on the number of visitors or on visiting hours.

Clearly, health care practitioners cannot be well versed in every custom or practice that may impinge on clinical management or affect a patient's behavior. Nor is it wise to stereotype patients and assume that everyone from a particular ethnic or cultural background will display a certain behavior or subscribe to certain beliefs and practices. It does make sense, however, for health care providers to make a systematic effort to learn about the cultural characteristics of the populations they serve, just as they do about other characteristics of their markets, and to educate caregivers about the need to understand and respect individual cultural beliefs.

Eliciting Patients' Culturally Based Beliefs

Clinicians at the Family Practice Residency program at the San Jose, California, Health Center follow a set of guidelines to improve cross-cultural communication about health with a diverse patient population (Berlin and Fowkes, 1983). These guidelines have been structured around the mnemonic acronym LEARN:

- *L*isten with sympathy and understanding to the patient's perception of the problem
- *E*xplain your perceptions of the problem
- *A*cknowledge and discuss the differences and similarities
- *R*ecommend treatment
- *N*egotiate agreement

While the traditional medical interview focuses on a patient's factual, subjective report of the onset, duration, and characteristics of symptoms, the LEARN approach shifts the focus to the patient's theoretical explanation of the reasons for the problem. The practitioner begins by asking such questions as "What do you feel may be causing your problem?" or "How do you feel the illness is affecting you?" or What do you feel might be of benefit?" to gain an understanding of the patient's explanatory model and preferences for treatment. The clinician then explains what the problem seems to be, from a biomedical point of view. At the same time, the practitioner acknowledges the patient's explanatory model, pointing out areas of agreement as well as potential conceptual conflicts. With the patient's involvement, the clinician recommends a treatment plan, trying to include culturally relevant approaches that will enhance its acceptability and negotiating with the patient to ensure that it is satisfactory. Most often, the patient's model does not create major therapeutic dilemmas and can be incorporated relatively easily into the health care plan. Clinicians have successfully incorporated this model into the structure of the clinical encounter and have reported improved communication, heightened awareness of cultural issues in medical care, and improved patient acceptance of treatment plans.

Formalized cultural assessment guides have also been recently developed for nurses. They generally aim to identify major cultural factors that may be important in working with patients from different cultural backgrounds. Tripp-Reimer, Brink, and Saunders (1984, p. 79) describe cultural assessment as a process of negotiation between client and professional in which each contributes important and relevant material and is treated as an equal. The assessment process has three stages. In the first stage, the nurse attempts to solicit information—in the person's own words—about the patient's background, including ethnicity and degree of affiliation with an ethnic or religious group, and about patterns of decision making, as well as anything else that may affect communication, such as language, styles of verbal and nonverbal communication, and norms of etiquette. In the second stage, the nurse tries to elicit the patient's specific reasons for seeking professional help, ideas about the illness, and views of previous and anticipated treatments. Similar to the first stage of the LEARN model, questions asked may include "What do you think has caused your problem?" or "What do you fear about your sickness?" and "What are the most important results you hope to receive from this treatment?" The third stage occurs after a nursing diagnosis has been made and specifically aims to uncover cultural factors that may influence intervention strategies. These may include the patient's feelings about the illness, how the patient thinks family and friends will react to the news of the illness, how the patient thinks someone in that condition is supposed to act, and what the patient is planning to do about the condition.

As in the LEARN model, negotiation between the patient's and the provider's explanatory models is essential, in order to improve the congruence between them. When the patient's health belief system is incorporated into the treatment plan, acceptance of the plan and compliance with therapeutic regimens improve (Fleming, 1989).

St. Mary's Hospital and Health Center in Tucson, Arizona, has also developed a program designed to recognize and respect the health belief systems of the Native American population it serves. The program began in 1984, at the suggestion of an Apache nurse who was distressed at the Anglo staff's failure to give the Indian patients the spiritual support they needed or the respect for their beliefs that they deserved. Following a series of educational workshops on Native American cultural traditions, the hospital set up a more formal program under the direction of a Comanche medicine man, formerly a National Traditional Indian Medicine Specialist from the Indian Health Service. The Traditional Indian Medicine Program offers St. Mary's Native American patients, on request, the medicine man's spiritual counseling and prayer services. It also welcomes other traditional healers on the patient units, and program staff ensure that their ceremonies are not interfered with. In addition, the hospital provides translation services for non-English speakers of Papago and Yaqui. The Traditional Indian Medicine Program also offers training for the hospital's nursing staff on the spiritual aspects of healing and sponsors conferences and workshops for staff of other hospitals on the applications of the program to other settings.

Involving Patients in Their Care:
Information, Communication, and Control

"I think different people have different expectations. . . . I think that maybe they [clinicians] should try to get into your head, first, and find out how involved you want to be." These words, spoken by a patient in one of our focus groups, conjure up the image of a clinician neatly and cleanly lifting the top of a patient's head to find an unequivocal answer to the question, "How involved do you want to be in your medical care?" Of course, in real-life medical encounters, patient and clinician must struggle through this question. They must tear down social, cultural, economic, and linguistic barriers, eliminate time constraints, and discard time-honored patterns of interaction.

Several researchers have tried to elucidate the characteristics that distinguish patients who want to be involved in their care from those who do not (Cassileth, Zupkis, and Sutton-Smith, 1980; Faden and others, 1981; Pendleton and House, 1984; Strull, Lo, and Charles, 1984). But the lack of consensus about what constitutes an "involved" or an "active" patient or about how such concepts should be measured makes it difficult to draw any general conclusions from this work. In fact, any effort to attach a global meaning to the concept of the "active" patient is bound to fail, since each patient defines "involvement" idiosyncratically. It may mean anything from asking a clinician a few questions during a visit to being a full partner in all aspects of clinical decision making.

Moreover, a patient's preference for involvement, however it is defined, is not static. Time, experience, and the course of illness can dramatically affect both the ability and the desire to participate. One patient in a focus group described the experience of his mother who, once active in managing her care, now wanted all medical decisions to be made for her. She had gotten to the point, he said, that "she really didn't want to know. She didn't care." Respecting patients' preferences therefore entails continual reassessment.

With these caveats in mind, let us now examine what we know about patients' preferences for involvement, how effectively those preferences have been respected, and what mechanisms exist that might enhance their participation and sense of control over the processes of care that affect them.

Information and Decision Making

Almost all patients wish to participate in their care to the extent that they want accurate, honest, and complete information about their illness, treatment options, and prognosis. Of the patients we interviewed on the Picker/Commonwealth national survey, 98 percent agreed that when there is more than one way to treat a medical problem, the choices should be discussed with the patient. It is also clear that many patients feel they are not receiving adequate information. Waitzkin (1985) found that patients are more dissatisfied about the information they receive from their physicians than about any other aspect of medical care, except high costs and waiting times. Moreover, clinicians tend to *underestimate* the extent to which patients want to know about and discuss alternative medical procedures and their risks and benefits (Faden and others, 1981; Strull, Lo, and Charles, 1984; Wetle, Levkoff, Cwikel, and Rosen, 1988). They also *overestimate* the amount of time they actually spend informing patients (Waitzkin, 1985).

While patients want medical information, they may hesitate to voice their questions and concerns. Some fall easily into the passive "sick role," a role characterized by an apparent lack of interest and involvement that may be fostered by the institutional environment. One patient we interviewed explained her own failure to query her caregivers: "I would like to know the possible side effects of any medicine I take. I didn't ask. I . . . felt pretty helpless and vulnerable and just didn't ask." Waterworth and Luker's (1990) findings from interviews with twelve medical patients of both sexes suggested that hospitalized patients, indeed, tend to "toe the line." The patients they interviewed were more concerned about doing "what is right" or pleasing the nurse than with taking part in decisions about their care. As one respondent explained, "I don't like asking too many questions, because if you ask too many questions you can get to be a bloody nuisance, and I think they know what they are doing."

Patients may also be inhibited by what Brody (1980) has described as the "information gap" between patients and clinicians. Patients are unlikely ever to have a clinical professional's facility with pathophysiological terms or concepts. They may find medical terminology intimidating and physiological functions mysterious. They may be afraid of demonstrating their ignorance by asking questions, or of receiving answers that only leave them baffled. Waitzkin (1985) has also shown that class-based differences in the "predisposition to seek and to offer information through verbal channels" can impede patient-physician communication, although patients of different social classes do not differ markedly in their desire for information. Silence on the part of the patients, then, does not always indicate lack of interest, and patients may need to be taught or led to ask questions, as one patient we interviewed suggested: "I don't think it should be totally up to the patient to ask the questions. . . . The patient doesn't know enough to ask the questions. So I think it's up to the caregiver to lead the patient, draw it out of the patient—'What are your concerns?' or 'What would you like to know?' "

Although most patients want to be informed about treatment options, the course of their illness, and the prospect of recovery, they do not necessarily want to take part in decisions about their treatment (Faden and others, 1981; Strull, Lo, and Charles, 1984). One focus-group patient made this clear, as he described his frustration getting information from his doctor: "[It was] not that I was going to tell him what to do or how to do anything. I'm not a doctor. I just wanted to know what he was doing and how he was coming along with it." Of the patients we surveyed nationally, only slightly more than half (57 percent) thought that a hospitalized patient should make decisions about medical care.

However, in examining the link between what he calls an "active patient orientation" and treatment outcomes, Schulman (1979) found that hypertensive patients who participated actively in decision making and treatment assumed more responsibility for their own care, used health resources more effectively, and were better able to control their blood pressure (Schulman, 1979; Steele, Blackwell, Gutmann, and Jackson, 1987). According to our survey findings, patients who do want to be involved in decisions about their care are more likely to be young (67 percent of those in the eighteen to forty year age group, as compared with 39 percent of those over sixty-five) and well educated (66 percent of those with a college degree, as opposed to 41 percent with no high school education). The same pattern appears in response to the survey question, "You should go along with your doctor's advice even when you think it is wrong," with age and education distinguishing those who deferred to their doctors from those who did not. Research elsewhere supports these findings (Cassileth, Zupkis, and Sutton-Smith, 1980; Pendleton and House, 1984; Strull, Lo, and Charles, 1984; Vertinsky, Thompson, and Uyeno, 1974), although it is not clear whether the observed phenomenon reflects differences in age or generational differences in attitudes toward authority.

Opening Channels of Communication

Lidz and his colleagues (1983) found the blurred lines of responsibility and internal communication between bureaucratic divisions and clinical specialties, especially in inpatient settings, to be a major barrier to informed consent. Patients often complain of having to repeat themselves to each new clinician involved in their case. As one patient said, "I . . . have a sense the doctors don't talk to each other. I have this sense that when I explain something . . . it stops right there." Traditional hospital structures and systems also limit patients' access to technical information, for example by keeping patients' records at nursing stations and restricting the use of hospital medical libraries to professional staff.

To enhance the quality of communication between clinicians and patients, some hospitals are experimenting with an "open-records" policy, allowing patients to read and write in their own charts (Altman, Reich, Kelley, and Rogers, 1980; Stevens, Stagg, and Mackay, 1977). The record alone is not likely to give patients all the information they want or need, nor will the language, medical abbreviations, and clinical information always be comprehensible to them. Some critics also fear that patients will be unnecessarily alarmed by what they read, especially if they do not understand it, and clinicians may object that the need to explain will increase the demands on their time. Defenders of the policy argue that it facilitates communication between physicians and pa-

tients precisely because it forces a dialogue. Patients on the Planetree Model Hospital Unit at California Pacific Medical Center, San
Francisco, are given access to their clinical records, invited to write
their own comments or concerns, and encouraged to discuss their
illness, course of treatment, and prognosis with their primary nurse
or physician. Planetree also offers patients access to a resource center,
where literature on virtually every medical condition or diagnostic
and therapeutic procedure is on hand or accessible—literature that
includes both lay and medical scientific publications.

Several researchers have also tried to find ways to help patients overcome the "passive patient" role and to become more
knowledgeable and active participants in their own care (Eisenthal,
Emery, Lazare, and Udin, 1979; Eisenthal, Koopman, and Lazare,
1983; Eisenthal and Lazare, 1976; Greenfield, Kaplan, and Ware,
1985; Langer and Rodin, 1976; Schulman, 1979; Stevens, Stagg, and
Mackay, 1977). Greenfield and others (1988) studied the effects of
giving patients with peptic ulcer disease short sessions, prior to each
visit with the doctor, to review their medical record and encourage
them to use the information to negotiate medical decisions. They
found that patients provided with such sessions were twice as effective in eliciting information from their physicians and reported
significantly fewer functional limitations as a result of their disease,
when compared with a control group not given the sessions. Eisenthal, Emery, Lazare, and Udin (1979) encourage the use of what
they call the "negotiated approach" to encourage patients to be
more assertive. They begin with the assumption that patients have
their own ideas about the nature, causes, severity, and consequences
of their illness and that they have expectations of their providers.
The clinician's role is to encourage the patient to voice these views
and expectations. Eisenthal and colleagues have found that use of
the "negotiated approach" correlates positively with patients' satisfaction with care, their sense of "feeling better," their ability to
achieve their desired disposition, and their adherence to medical
recommendations (Eisenthal and Lazare, 1976; Eisenthal, Koopman, and Lazare, 1983).

Autonomy and Control

One of the most common and disturbing sensations reported by
patients in our focus groups was an overwhelming feeling of help-

lessness while they were in the hospital, a loss of a sense of autonomy and control. As one patient explained it, "In the role of the patient, you are once again stripped of your control, regardless of how good the hospital is, and I think that's the biggest issue that I've had with being sick." For most sick people at some times, a certain degree of enforced passivity is both necessary and welcome. As one patient said, "I wanted to just be a patient and lie there and be taken care of." Beyond that point, however, it inhibits their recovery and affronts their dignity. One older woman in our focus group spoke of how simple things like being able to take a shower by herself or walk around the hospital made her feel less a victim of her illness and more like the independent person she once was.

Yet the traditional rules and regulations and standard operating procedures of most hospitals almost demand that patients be passive, submissive, and more or less inanimate. They require patients to be escorted by wheelchair, for example, when they can walk by themselves; they place strict limits on the number of visitors allowed and the hours of visitation; they discourage and sometimes prohibit patients from performing even limited medical tasks for themselves, such as changing dressings or taking charge of their own medications. Patients who comply submissively with "the system" are deemed "good" patients; those who challenge well-established hospital routines are seen as deviant, uncooperative, "problem" patients (Raps, Peterson, and Jonas, 1982). These expectations may be so routine a part of hospital life that they are hardly questioned by either patients or caregivers. One patient interviewed by Waterworth and Luker (1990, p. 972), for example, was asked what adjustments he had made in coming to the hospital. "Nothing really," he replied, "except do as I'm told. There's no force, they haven't forced you into any adjustment whatsoever except that you obey the rules. If they want more blood, they take more blood."

Gradually, hospitals are changing and finding ways to allow patients more control over medical and nonmedical aspects of their hospital care. Two of the most publicized experiments in changing hospital routines at the unit level are the Planetree Model Hospital Unit at California Pacific Medical Center in San Francisco and the Cooperative Care Unit at New York University Medical Center in New York. At Planetree, nurses do their best to schedule tests, procedures, meals, and so forth to suit the patients rather than the hospital bureaucracy. They will request later appointment times for patients who like to sleep in the morning, for example, or ask early-arriving laboratory technicians to come back later. Planetree patients are also allowed to participate in or manage much of their own medical care, with the help of friends or family members. In practice, the extent of their participation is limited by the degree of skill or training required and their own motivation. Many patients do take charge of their own medications, dressing changes, and the like, but others show no interest, and their wishes are respected.

At Coop Care, meals are taken in a central, communal dining room, where patients select food cafeteria style, instead of having preselected meals delivered on trays to their rooms. Wherever possible, Coop Care instructs each patient in a program of Self-Administered Medication. Once they have demonstrated to the consulting pharmacist's satisfaction that they can identify each medicine, know what it is for, and understand how and when it is to be administered, patients administer and chart their own medications. Further, patients at Coop Care wear street clothes, rather than hospital garb, on the unit, and they are distinguished only by the identification badges they are required to wear. They are free to come and go from their rooms or to visit the lounge or dining area. Coop Care patients also have more control over certain daily routines—when to go to sleep, when to wake up, when and what to eat, and where to go.

Understanding and Respecting Patients' Therapeutic Goals

"[The physicians] said I might have a little time. They were right. I could have had the treatments, but they didn't hold out any hope except maybe for a little delay. And there's all that appalling nastiness of losing your hair, and the people I've known who took those treatments were sick all the time. I decided I'd rather be intact for whatever time I was given" (Stegner, 1987, p. 290). Historically, medical decision making was the exclusive province of clinicians—ideally, a physician long known to the patient and family, whose trust was well established. Today, while the technical possibilities expand even at the margins of life, the physician in charge may have little or no prior history with that patient or family. Under the circumstances, clinicians want to rely on scientific data to dictate a course of action. But how compelling is science as a basis for clinical decision making? How does one weigh the advantages of chemotherapy, in the apparently terminal case depicted in the quotation above, against its "appalling nastiness?" What happens when the evidence is ambiguous, or science dictates a course of action at odds with what a patient wants? Here, we examine some of the practical implications of incorporating the patient's perspective into clinical decision making.

Therapy That Suits the Patient

At one of our site visits, we heard the story of a feisty woman in her seventies recovering from hip surgery who showed up for physical therapy wearing spike heels. When the therapists objected, telling her it was too dangerous, that she might fall and injure herself, the woman countered that she had *always* worn high heels and vowed not to leave the hospital until she could walk out in her heels. No doubt, if she had been a famous sports figure, she would have had less trouble overcoming her caregivers' cautious skepticism about treatment limitations. But what if she had not been so feisty? Would they have tried as they did to help her, or would they have dismissed her expectations as unimportant and unrealistic?

Clinicians who take patients' therapeutic goals seriously are more willing to take the time and effort to try to meet their needs. The Mayo Clinic and its affiliated hospitals have achieved some remarkable successes in equipping many chronically ill patients to maintain an independent existence, away from the clinic. One such patient who lives with Crohn's disease has been able to rely entirely on total parenteral nutrition for twelve years, even when traveling for his job as a marketing representative for a computer company.

In Whose "Best Interest"?

The remarkable achievements of medical technology over the past few decades have created unprecedented opportunities to save and prolong life or forestall death. But they have also created unprece-

dented ethical dilemmas. Is the quality of the lives that are prolonged worth the human cost, even to those who are saved? The
stakes are dramatic enough in the extreme cases that few people
would ask doctors to shoulder the burden of decision making by
themselves. Patients and providers alike look for ways to make the
patients' wishes known, even when they cannot speak for themselves, through such devices as living wills and advance directives.

But everyday clinical practice is not so dramatic, and the
stakes may not be so apparent. Lidz and his colleagues found that
most physicians believe that there is one preferred treatment option,
in most cases, and that the patient's health would be jeopardized if
an alternative were chosen. As a result, the physicians they observed
rarely discussed alternatives with their patients or solicited their
opinions; rather, they told patients what was going to be done and
the reasons for doing it (Lidz and others, 1983). When they do discuss alternatives, health care practitioners may exaggerate the benefits of the "desirable" option or the hazards of the "undesirable"
one (Forrow, Wartman, and Brock, 1988). One patient we interviewed, who resisted taking prescribed blood pressure medication
after childbirth because she was worried about its effect on her
psyche and her nursing child, described being warned that she
might "drop dead of a stroke" if she did not take it. This patient,
like most, needed time not only to come to terms with unwelcome
information, but to process it in light of her parallel concerns about
her own health, her child's health, and her ability to function effectively as a new mother.

In fact, patients and clinicians often have different criteria for
assessing the desirability or efficacy of alternative treatments.
McNeil and her associates found, for example, that when healthy,
knowledgeable, and informed volunteers were presented a hypothetical choice between radiation therapy and surgery to treat cancer of
the larynx, 20 percent chose radiation in order to preserve their
speech, even though it was associated with a much lower survival
rate (McNeil, Weichselbaum, and Pauker, 1981). Forrow and his
colleagues have also observed that for some hypertensive patients,
a small decrease in the risk of future mortality or morbidity may not
be worth the burdensome side effects of long-term hypertension
therapy. And yet physicians often tend to label such patients non-

compliant, to view their concerns as barriers to overcome rather than as rational and legitimate contraindications to medical intervention (Forrow, Wartman, and Brock, 1988; Conrad, 1987). Choices that medical professionals perceive as irrational may be based on informed and sound reasoning in line with patients' own values.

Incorporating Patients' Preferences into Clinical Decisions

Practicing clinicians have always understood that medical decision making is as much art as it is science. They rely increasingly on "hard" scientific data from physical examinations and laboratory tests to understand pathophysiological processes and establish clinical diagnoses and on the results of statistically controlled clinical trials to judge treatment efficacy. But scientific evidence is often limited and ambiguous (Kassirer and Pauker, 1981). And clinicians' ability to manage patient care and to anticipate the outcome of treatment *in practice* depends as much, or more, on "soft" information about patients' attitudes, preferences, and personal idiosyncrasies (Feinstein, 1983).

Historically, intuition and experience have guided practitioners in the art of medical practice, but researchers in recent years have tried to develop new decision-making models that incorporate contingencies, uncertainties, and individual values to improve the efficacy of clinical decisions (Kassirer, Moskowitz, Lau, and Pauker, 1987; Eraker, 1982; Eraker, Kirscht, and Becker, 1984). Clinical "decision analysis" entails, first, mapping out the logical sequence of a decision-making process, in much the way a computer programmer might do. Each decision "node" (or point at which a choice must be made) is identified, along with all of the alternative choices at each node and all of the potential outcomes of each choice together with the statistical probabilities of their occurrence. The result is a decision "tree," whose branches represent all of the possible combinations of choices and outcomes. Patients then decide the relative value (or "utility") of each possible outcome, based on their own individual preferences. Presumably, then, the "best" decision in any case is the one that has the best chance of maximizing the patient's utility, given intermediate probabilities.

Applying the principles of decision analysis to real clinical situations is difficult in practice. Patients may not know, for example, what "value" they would assign to outcomes entailing pain, disability, or unpleasant side effects when they have no experience of them (Eraker, 1982; Eraker, Kirscht, and Becker, 1984). Moreover, their expressed preferences may vary depending on how the question is framed (Kahneman and Tversky, 1984) or on the methodology used to assign numerical values to their utilities (Read and others, 1984; Kahneman and Tversky, 1984; Eraker, 1982). Any given decision analytical model may also overestimate the likelihood of a favorable outcome, because it fails to take into account the system and human errors that unexpectedly, but inevitably, occur along the way (Palmer, Strain, Rothrock, and Hsu, 1983). Nonetheless, this approach to modeling clinical decisions helps identify the areas of scientific uncertainty, clarify the alternatives, and elucidate the value judgments that must come into play at every stage of the decision-making process.

Summary

Understanding and respecting patients' values, preferences, and expressed needs is the foundation of patient-centered care. Although disease processes may be described in physiological terms, illness and the experience of illness can only be described as a social and cultural phenomenon. Culture—in the broad sense of the word that includes not only ethnicity but also class, gender, and other social attributes—affects how patients understand their illness, how they respond to it, how they communicate about it, and how it affects their lives. Even when patient and provider come from similar social backgrounds, the disparity in their respective understanding of an illness can be jarring, once it is apparent. It is all the more so when the social or cultural distance between them is larger. The development of appropriate and effective therapeutic strategies entails a negotiated understanding between the culture of biomedicine, within which health care providers work, and the patient's cultural experience of illness.

Patients vary in their willingness to participate in the culture of biomedicine or take part in their own care. Sickness often makes people more passive than they would otherwise be, content simply to let others take care of them and make decisions for them. They may therefore quite willingly submit to the ministrations of health care professionals. On the other hand, the institutional routines and the technologies that the biomedical world has created often *require* patients to be passive and submissive, making their attempts at assertiveness or control appear disruptive. But patients who are able to take a more active part in their care may have a better recovery. Whether or not they want to know every statistic related to their case or take part in clinical decisions, almost every patient wants honest, accurate information about what clinicians think is wrong with them, what they plan to do about it, and what outcomes they expect. And yet health care providers routinely misjudge how much their patients want to know or do. Providers need to reexamine the institutional structures and routine practices that foster a needless, perhaps even harmful, dependency in patients.

Providers may be reluctant to inform patients fully about treatment options, side effects, or outcomes, or to encourage them to take part in decisions, for fear that they will make a decision that is not in their best interest. But informed, rational patients may have a different view of their "best interest" than the professionals who care for them. They may have a different idea as to what constitutes an acceptable risk, a tolerable side effect, or an unavoidable disability. Although the mathematical rigor required of full-scale decision analysis may not be practical in everyday clinical practice, it offers a conceptual approach to clinical decision making that makes it possible for clinician and patient together to clarify options, outcomes, uncertainties, and values.

Suggestions for Improvement

- Educate staff about the health beliefs, practices, and mores of specific ethnic and cultural groups in your patient population.
- Develop comprehensive planning focused on the needs of cultural, as well as diagnostic, groups of patients.
- Develop nursing and clinical interview protocols that elicit patients' perceptions about their illness and their expectations of treatment.

- Develop explicit and culturally appropriate expectations and standards regarding staff behavior with patients—for example, forms of address, knocking on doors, rules of propriety.
- Educate staff to ask, not assume: to ask patients what they want to know, to suggest questions that patients might have, to ask patients if they understand, and so on.
- Consider giving patients access to medical records, if they want it, and make sure knowledgeable staff are available to encourage questions and to talk with them about the records.
- Reexamine institutional routines that force patients into passive compliance; wherever possible, let patients do and control as much as they can on their own.
- Educate staff to ask, not assume, how therapeutic decisions affect patients' lives and what patients' preferences would be among alternative treatments and outcomes.
- Educate clinical staff to negotiate therapeutic strategies with patients.

References

Altman, J., Reich, P., Kelley, M., and Rogers, M. "Patients Who Read Their Hospital Charts." *New England Journal of Medicine*, 1980, *302*, 169–171.

Baron, R. J. "Bridging Clinical Distance: An Empathic Rediscovery of the Known." *Journal of Medical Philosophy*, 1981, *6*, 5–23.

Baron, R. J. "An Introduction to Medical Phenomenology: I Can't Hear You While I'm Listening." *Annals of Internal Medicine*, 1985, *103*, 606–611.

Berlin, E. A., and Fowkes, W. C. "A Teaching Framework for Cross-Cultural Health Care." *Western Journal of Medicine*, 1983, *139*, 934–938.

Brody, D. S. "The Patient's Role In Clinical Decision-Making." *Annals of Internal Medicine*, 1980, *93*, 718–722.

Cassell, E. J. "Treating Patients for Both is the Healer's Art: Illness and Disease." *Hastings Center Report*, 1976, *6*, 27–37.

Cassell, E. J. "The Nature of Suffering and the Goals of Medicine." *New England Journal of Medicine*, 1982, *306*, 639–645.

Cassell, E. J. "Life as a Work of Art." *Hastings Center Report,* 1984, *14,* 35–37.

Cassileth, B. R., Zupkis, R. V., and Sutton-Smith, K. "Information and Participation Preferences Among Cancer Patients." *Annals of Internal Medicine,* 1980, *92,* 832–836.

Conrad, P. "The Noncompliant Patient in Search of Autonomy." *Hastings Center Report,* 1987, *17,* 15–17.

Eisenberg, L. "Disease and Illness." *Culture, Medicine, and Psychiatry,* 1977, *1,* 9–23.

Eisenthal, S., Emery, R., Lazare, A., and Udin, H. "Adherence and the Negotiated Approach to Patienthood." *Archives of General Psychiatry,* 1979, *36,* 393–398.

Eisenthal, S., Koopman, C., and Lazare, A. "Process Analysis of Two Dimensions of the Negotiated Approach in Relation to Satisfaction in the Initial Interview." *Journal of Nervous and Mental Disorders,* 1983, *171,* 49–54.

Eisenthal, S., and Lazare, A. "Evaluation of the Initial Interview in a Walk-In Clinic." *Journal of Nervous and Mental Disorders,* 1976, *162,* 169–176.

Eraker, S. A. "How Decisions Are Reached: Physician and Patient." *Annals of Internal Medicine,* 1982, *97,* 262–268.

Eraker, S. A., Kirscht, J. P., and Becker, M. H. "Understanding and Improving Patient Compliance." *Annals of Internal Medicine,* 1984, *100,* 259–268.

Faden, R. R., and others. "Disclosure of Information to Patients in Medical Care." *Medical Care,* 1981, *14,* 718–733.

Feinstein, A. R. "An Additional Basic Science for Clinical Medicine. 1: The Constraining Fundamental Paradigms." *Annals of Internal Medicine,* 1983, *99,* 393–397.

Fleming, J. "Meeting the Challenge of Culturally Diverse Populations." *Pediatric Nursing,* 1989, *15,* 566, 634–648.

Forrow, L., Wartman, S. A., and Brock, D. W. "Science, Ethics, and the Making of Clinical Decisions: Implications for Risk Factor Intervention." *Journal of the American Medical Association,* 1988, *259,* 3161–3167.

Greenfield, S., Kaplan, S. H., and Ware, J. E., Jr. "Expanding Patient Involvement in Care: Effects on Patient Outcome." *Annals of Internal Medicine,* 1985, *102,* 520–528.

Greenfield, S., and others. "Patients' Participation in Medical Care: Effects on Blood Sugar Control and Quality of Life in Diabetes." *Journal of General Internal Medicine*, 1988, *3*, 448–457.

Hautman, M. A. "Folk Health and Illness Beliefs." *Nurse Practitioner*, 1979, *4*, 23–24.

Helman, C. G. *Culture, Health, and Illness.* (2nd ed.) London: Butterworth, 1990.

Kahneman, D., and Tversky, A. "Choices, Values, and Frames." *American Psychologist*, 1984, *39*, 341–350.

Kassirer, J. P., and Pauker, S. G. "The Toss-Up." *New England Journal of Medicine*, 1981, *305*, 1467–1469.

Kassirer, J. P., Moskowitz, A. J., Lau, J., and Pauker, S. G. "Decision Analysis: A Progress Report." *Annals of Internal Medicine*, 1987, *106*, 275–291.

Kleinman, A., Eisenberg, L., and Good, B. "Culture, Illness, and Care: Clinical Lessons from Anthropologic and Cross-Cultural Research." *Annals of Internal Medicine*, 1978, *88*, 251–258.

Langer, E. J., and Rodin, J. "The Effects of Choice and Enhanced Personal Responsibility for the Aged: A Field Experiment in an Institutional Setting." *Journal of Personality and Social Psychology*, 1976, *34*, 191–198.

Lidz, C. W., and others. "Barriers to Informed Consent." *Annals of Internal Medicine*, 1983, *99*, 539–543.

Lorber, J. "Good Patients and Problem Patients: Conformity and Deviance in a General Hospital." *Journal of Health and Social Behavior*, 1975, *16*, 213–225.

McNeil, B. J., Weichselbaum, R., and Pauker, S. G. "Speech and Survival: Tradeoffs Between Quality and Quantity of Life in Laryngeal Cancer." *New England Journal of Medicine*, 1981, *305*, 982–987.

Palmer, R. H., Strain, R., Rothrock, J. K., and Hsu, L. "Evaluations of Operational Failures in Clinical Decision Making." *Medical Decision Making*, 1983, *3*, 299–310.

Pendleton, L., and House, W. C. "Preferences for Treatment Approaches in Medical Care: College Students Versus Diabetic Outpatients." *Medical Care*, 1984, *22*, 644–646.

Qureshi, B. *Transcultural Medicine.* Dordrecht, Holland: Kluwer Academic Publishers, 1989.

Raps, C. S., Peterson, C., and Jonas, M. "Patient Behavior in Hospitals: Helplessness, Reactance, or Both?" *Journal of Personality and Social Psychology*, 1982, *42*, 1036-1041.

Read, J. L., and others. "Preferences for Health Outcomes: Comparison of Assessment Methods." *Medical Decision Making*, 1984, *4*, 315-329.

Rothenburger, R. L. "Transcultural Nursing." *AORN Journal*, 1990, *51*, 1349-1363.

Schulman, B. A. "Active Patient Orientation and Outcomes in Hypertensive Treatment." *Medical Care*, 1979, *17*, 267-280.

Snow, L. F. "Folk Medical Beliefs and Their Implications for Care of Patients: A Review Based on Studies Among Black Americans." *Annals of Internal Medicine*, 1974, *81*, 82-96.

Spector, R. E. *Cultural Diversity in Health and Illness.* New York: Appleton-Century-Crofts, 1979.

Steele, D., Blackwell, B., Gutmann, M., and Jackson, T. "The Activated Patient: Dogma, Dream, or Desideratum?" *Patient Education and Counseling*, 1987, *10*, 3-23.

Stegner, W. *Crossing to Safety.* New York: Penguin Books, 1987.

Stevens, D. P., Stagg, R., and Mackay, I. R. "What Happens When Hospitalized Patients See Their Own Records?" *Annals of Internal Medicine*, 1977, *86*, 474-477.

Strull, W. M., Lo, B., and Charles, G. "Do Patients Want to Participate in Medical Decision Making?" *Journal of the American Medical Association*, 1984, *252*, 2990-2994.

Tripp-Reimer, T., Brink, P. J., and Saunders, J. M. "Cultural Assessment: Content and Process." *Nursing Outlook*, 1984, *32*, 78-82.

Vertinsky, I. B., Thompson, W. A., and Uyeno, D. "Measuring Consumer Desire for Participation in Clinical Decision Making." *Health Services Research*, 1974, *9*, 121-134.

Waitzkin, H. "Information Giving in Medical Care." *Journal of Health and Social Behavior*, 1985, *26*, 81-101.

Waterworth, S., and Luker, K. A. "Reluctant Collaborators: Do Patients Want to Be Involved in Decisions Concerning Their Care?" *Journal of Advanced Nursing*, 1990, *15*, 971-976.

Wetle, T., Levkoff, S., Cwikel, J., and Rosen, A. "Nursing Home

Resident Participation in Medical Decisions: Perceptions and Preferences." *Gerontologist,* 1988, *28,* 32–38.

Zola, I. K. "Culture and Symptoms: An Analysis of Patients' Presenting Complaints." *American Sociological Review,* 1966, *31,* 615–630.

3

Coordinating Care
and Integrating Services

Margaret Gerteis

When we asked the patients in our focus groups to describe what mattered to them most while they were in the hospital, one of the things they mentioned most often was the importance of feeling that they were in competent hands. If they had that feeling, then they could relax—at least as much as their circumstances would allow. If not, they were worried, fearful, tense, on guard—or else they relied on their family and friends to be on guard for them. How do patients make such judgments? What makes them trust the competence of some caregivers and not others? How do they decide whether or not they are in "good hands"?

Health care professionals are sometimes uneasy at the thought of patients judging the quality of their care. Patients do not have the expertise necessary to assess quality, and what they base their judgments on has little to do with real quality, the argument goes (Lebow, 1974; Steiber, 1988; Press, 1984; Omachonu, 1990). By that reasoning, if we earnestly want to promote better health care, we should pay more attention to objective measures of quality and less attention to what patients think. Undoubtedly, patients' judgments about quality and competence are influenced by such things as the training and experience of the professionals who tend them, their ability to diagnose and treat what ails them, the availability of up-to-date equipment, and other more-or-less tangible features of technical quality. Whether or not patients are good at sensing such

things, there is no question that these aspects of quality are best
assessed through objective measures and standards. And health care
providers will always have an ethical responsibility to see that care
meets these standards, regardless of what patients think or notice—
just as engineers, mechanics, and pilots are responsible for the safety
and performance of an aircraft, whatever the passengers might have
to say about the airline's operations.

Still, we contend that the way patients judge the competence
and quality of their care *does* matter. It matters, first of all, because
whether or not it jibes with professional assessments, what patients
believe to be true will determine how they act. If they do not trust
a provider or a facility, they may not follow through with recommended treatment, or they may decide to go somewhere else (Inguanzo and Harju, 1985). Patients' perceptions also matter because
they offer firsthand information about health care delivery that may
not be available through other means. As the end points of delivery
systems, patients are eyewitnesses to how those systems work. The
significance of this vantage point becomes clear when one probes
beyond global statements to ask patients what, in particular, contributes to their reported feelings of confidence and trust, or its
absence. Much of what they comment about has little to do with
professional skills or qualifications or adherence to technical standards and protocols. They speak, instead, of "efficiency" and "well-
oiled machines"—judgments that have more to do with how well
care seems to be coordinated and integrated in a total system. And
it is precisely this phenomenon that can be hard to document
objectively.

In this chapter, we address this dimension of health care
quality—the coordination and integration of care—and the factors
that influence patients' perceptions of it. We look, in turn, at three
distinct tasks of coordination unique to the environment of hospitals and health care facilities (borrowing from Koeck and Levitt,
1990):

1. Coordination of clinical care—both the "horizontal" integra-
    tion of specialties and subspecialties and the "vertical" integra-
    tion of professional hierarchies

2. Coordination of clinical support services—diagnostic and therapeutic support services
3. Coordination of the delivery of patient care—nursing and ancillary "front-line" patient care

Coordination of Clinical Care

We turn our attention first to problems and potential solutions related to the coordination of clinical care.

Problems

Rarely, these days—and hardly ever in hospitals—is a single physician solely responsible for the clinical care of a patient. More often, a multiplicity of players is involved in clinical observation, decision making, and treatment, each with a different measure of status and area of expertise (Freidson, 1970). This situation can be confusing to patients and caregivers alike.

Who's in charge? Amid the confusion of specialists, subspecialists, doctors, nurses, and interns that a patient is likely to encounter in an acute care facility, the first question that must be answered is, "Who's in charge?" The relationships and lines of authority among the players are especially diffuse in academic health centers, where there are both lateral peer relations among specialists or consultants involved in a case and a set of hierarchical relations among attending physicians, senior and junior residents, medical students, and nurses and other nonphysicians involved in clinical care. In her pioneering study of medical and surgical wards in a large teaching hospital, sociologist Rose Coser (1958, 1962) observed more than thirty years ago the complex and subtle differences not only in formal structures, but in actual patterns of decision making—differences that even members of the clinical team picked up only in practice. On the surgical ward, she observed, relations among the attending surgeons, residents, and nurses appeared to be quite collegial: they all tended to talk and joke with one another, without respect to formal lines of authority, and all participated in rounds, contributing their various observations, opinions, and suggestions. But in practice, it was the attending

surgeon or chief surgical resident who made all the decisions. On
the medical ward, the opposite was true: relations among members
of the team were more polite, formal, and rigidly hierarchical, with
the attending or chief physician dominating rounds, residents answering only direct questions put to them, and the nurses doing
little more than wheeling the charts around. But in this case, most
of the real authority over day-to-day clinical decision making was
delegated down the line to the junior residents or interns.

If it takes a sociologist or a seasoned participant to figure out
this pattern of relations, consider how bewildering it is to the patient who confronts, as one patient described it, "a slew of progressively younger and more nervous people coming in and examining
me." One medical patient we interviewed, who had been hospitalized with pneumonia, complained of having "two doctors" examine her simultaneously, one listening to one side of her chest, the
other listening to the other side. The "doctors" were most likely
residents engaging in what is popularly known as "double team-
ing," or perhaps medical students practicing the art of auscultation.
In any case, nobody explained to the patient who they were or what
they were doing, and she was left wondering at the bizarre division
of labor that would have each doctor take a different lung. "I was
not impressed," she remarked.

Not knowing who is in charge, patients may conclude that
no one is. Of the patients we interviewed in the Picker/Common-
wealth national survey, 15 percent believed that there was no one
particular doctor in charge of their care while they were in the
hospital. The proportion so reporting rose to 20 percent among
patients hospitalized in an academic health center—nearly twice as
many as believed that to be the case in nonteaching hospitals (11
percent). The problem is not limited to academic health centers,
however, even though they may represent the most confusing environments. Many patients will confront an array of specialists and
consultants when they enter the hospital. Moreover, even if they
have one primary care physician they see regularly, they may not
be treated by that doctor in the hospital, especially if they are admitted for surgery. Of the patients we surveyed nationally, 87 percent reported having a "regular doctor," but only 54 percent were
cared for by that doctor while they were in the hospital; among

surgical patients, only 43 percent saw their regular doctor in the hospital.

Moreover, the patterns of authority among members of the clinical team may shift during the course of an illness or a hospitalization in ways that may not be obvious to the patient. One oncology patient (a clinician herself) hospitalized for a mastectomy soon after she was diagnosed with breast cancer was surprised to learn that the oncologist, and not the surgeon, was the "quarterback" of her clinical team, since it was the surgeon who had played the more prominent role at that early stage of her treatment. Journalist Joyce Wadler (1992) was similarly confused by the "growing group of specialists" she confronted after being diagnosed with breast cancer: "What this disease needs . . . is a contractor," she concluded "—or at least one room where we could get all the doctors together."

How effectively do clinicians communicate and work with one another? Wadler's desire to get all her doctors together in one room reflects another common frustration among patients: a sense that their clinicians do not talk to each other. Patients in focus groups speaking about their hospital experiences, and many others we interviewed, often complained of being asked to give the same information over and over again. Of course, there may be good reasons for doctors and nurses to ask questions again and again— when a consultant wants to elicit significant details, for example, or hear a patient describe symptoms, firsthand. However, when patients sense that members of the clinical team are not passing along critical pieces of information to one another, they are not inspired with confidence in the team's effectiveness. Sometimes the patient's perceptions are accurate (Wessen, 1958). One participant in a patient focus group, who had been hospitalized a second time for a myocardial infarction and angioplasty, described his frustration at his doctors' failure to consult his earlier medical records from another institution: "When they came around in rounds, I said, 'Did you get my records from the other hospital?' And they said, 'Uh, no,' and they scooted out, the whole group. They never got them! So, when I was let out and I knew I was gonna have to come back in, I said, 'I'm gonna get my records and I'm gonna bring them in with me, 'cause nobody seems to bother. It's not important to them.' "

The diffusion of clinical responsibility complicates both the task of communication among the various members of the clinical team and the flow of information. Lidz and his colleagues (1983) in a study they conducted for the Institute of Medicine, found that one of the biggest informational barriers in hospitals is confusion among the team members themselves as to who is responsible for communicating what to whom. Clearly, communication breakdowns, quite apart from the fact that they disturb patients or leave them uninformed, can seriously affect the quality of clinical care. In 52 percent of the cases from pediatric group practices examined by Palmer and her co-investigators, for example, clinicians failed to follow up abnormal test results according to well-established and accepted criteria because of "operational failures" in the decision-making sequence—failures that included information not going to the right people, ambiguous lines of responsibility, and other system and "human" errors (Palmer, Strain, Rothrock, and Hsu, 1983). Another major study found that the quality of coordination and communication among members of clinical teams on intensive care units accounted for significant variations in outcomes among the units (Knaus, Draper, Wagner, and Zimmerman, 1986).

Patients are often central witnesses to such system failures. What they may see is that the people taking care of them are uninformed; that efforts are needlessly duplicated; that procedures are delayed, tasks left undone. Of the patients we surveyed nationally, between 10 and 11 percent reported that things were either done that should not have been done or that the reverse was true at some point in their hospitalization. Again, patients in academic health centers were more likely to report such failures (13–14 percent), as were patients with higher levels of education and income (13–16 percent).

Do members of the clinical team deliver a consistent set of messages to the patient and family? Patients' perceptions of the quality of their clinical care will also be colored by the consistency of the messages they receive from various members of the clinical team. Do they seem to be in accord with one another, or are there obvious points of discord? Is the patient left with a clear understanding of treatment alternatives or bewildered by conflicting opinions and advice? Of course, the situation is complicated by the fact that patients are not merely passive receivers of the messages that clinicians craft and deliver. Patients, too, acting out of uncertainty, fear, or confusion, ask the same questions of many different people. They may want to reassure themselves that no one is keeping anything from them—a fear commonly expressed in the patient focus groups, they may want to "test" their caregivers, or they may want to fish for the answer that most satisfies them (McIntosh, 1974). As one former surgical patient told us, "I had two doctors. They both came to see me daily and they both explained everything to me daily. I'd ask one a question, and I'd ask the other—or I'd play one against the other. If I didn't like the answer, I went to the other, and eventually I would get the answer I wanted."

Whether or not they receive a consistent set of messages will depend, in part, on how well members of the clinical team communicate with each other. But it will also depend on the patient's and the team's ability to recognize the appropriate spokesperson, depending on the nature of the information to be communicated— and that may not be obvious either to the patient or to other members of the team. Lidz and others (1983) observed that responsibility for informing patients on the cardiology ward was so diffuse that it was sometimes overlooked entirely and that responsibility for decision making was so ambiguous that many patients did not know where to turn for information. Even patients who have a sophisticated understanding of their illness may be constitutionally and emotionally unequal to the task of sorting through for themselves differing opinions and pieces of advice. The late Dr. Franz Ingelfinger was barraged by "well-intentioned but contradictory advice" from physician friends throughout the country, after he was diagnosed with adenocarcinoma. "As a result," he recalled, "not only I but my wife, my son and daughter-in-law (both doctors) . . . became increasingly confused and emotionally distraught. Finally, when the pangs of indecision had become nearly intolerable, one wise physician friend said, 'What you need is a doctor' " (Ingelfinger, 1980, p. 1510).

Patients may also be confused by conflicting messages coming from outside their present system of care. When they have been frustrated or disappointed by one set of providers, they often shop around. How are they to process dissenting second and third opinions, variations in treatment protocols, or the advice of alternative therapeutic practitioners? The improvisational comedienne and actress Gilda Radner, in her frustrating search for the cause and a cure for a debilitating array of symptoms, turned (like many others in her predicament) to holistic healers, in addition to her regular doctors. She described her resulting state of confusion: "I began to wonder how to please so many people. Do I take the magnesium citrate? What about the coffee enema? Do I do both? Do I do the abdominal massage or the colonic? Do I tell the doctors about each other?" (Radner, 1989, p. 67).

Solutions

As the foregoing discussion suggests, coordinating clinical care, from the patient's perspective, entails both clarifying the lines of authority and responsibility internally among the members of the clinical team and conveying that information to the patient. Much of the confusion we encountered among patients could have been alleviated if someone had simply explained to them who the players were and what their roles and responsibilities were. Someone might also have told the patients we surveyed, for example, which doctor, among the many they saw, was actually in charge of their care. The chief executive officer of Parkland Hospital in Dallas, Texas, is tackling this problem by posting photographs of team members on each clinical unit and by giving each patient a card listing the names, titles, and functions of the team members assigned to the patient's care.

It also helps if there is one readily identifiable person who can act as the patient's guide and interpreter. In many cases, a physician, a nurse, or some other knowledgeable "insider" will assume the role voluntarily or fall into it serendipitously. In others, hospital managers who recognize the need will assign the job explicitly. At the University of Chicago Hospitals, for example, a patient "special services" representative, whose job is to shepherd patients referred from outside the area through the system, from admission to discharge, may help demystify the organizational complexities as well as run interference for the patient. At least part of the rationale behind primary nursing is also to give patients a central point of access and information. The effectiveness of any designated spokesperson, however, will be limited by the scope of that person's knowledge, status, and authority. A spokesperson who is not a fully participating member of the clinical team, for instance, will have limited understanding of clinical issues, and will necessarily defer to others on such questions. Moreover, no designated spokesperson will be able to resolve a patient's confusion or build a patient's trust in the quality of care, if the underlying problems of diffuse authority, ambiguous lines of responsibility, and communication failures remain. It takes someone with recognized status and clinical authority to be the integrative force on the clinical team.

Without the active involvement of physicians and especially of the physician in charge, the success of any mechanism designed to integrate clinical care in a hospital or health care organization will be limited. Yet traditionally, the relationship between doctors and the institutions they and their patients depend on has been indirect and ambiguous. Perhaps for this reason, the best examples of clinical integration are found in those institutions organized according to a physician staff model. At the Mayo Clinic, for example, there is no question as to who "the doctor" is, in the sense Dr. Ingelfinger implied. There, all clinical responsibility—including the initial physical examination and workup, ordering of tests and procedures, and all clinical decision making—rests exclusively with the doctor to whom each patient is referred on the initial visit. Almost nothing is delegated. That one physician is the sole repository for all relevant clinical information and the only person responsible for communicating with the patient and family. The lines of authority and information flow are unequivocal.

Hospitals organized along more traditional lines have also had some noteworthy success in improving the coordination and integration of clinical care around particular disease categories—especially when physicians' interests in maintaining referrals in those areas coincide with the hospital's interest in developing or maintaining potential sources of patients. The University of Chicago Hospitals, for example, have been able to establish such an identity of interests around certain areas of tertiary care, and they have vastly improved their physicians' involvement with the organization and delivery of clinical services and processes of internal and external communication. Other hospitals have made similar achievements in their efforts to integrate a broad array of inpatient and outpatient services in such specialty areas as oncology, heart disease, and obstetrics, as part of a larger marketing strategy.

One thing that has hampered hospitals in their attempts to involve physicians in other such integrative efforts, however, is that to many doctors, "quality improvement," "quality review," and "quality assessment" may connote a thinly disguised institutional effort to control or interfere with the way they practice, usually for the purpose of controlling costs. Evaluating the performance of individual doctors against established standards or norms can further antagonize them and reinforce their sense of an underlying *dis*harmony of interests (Wennberg, 1990). The more recent tendency characteristic of continuous quality improvement to focus on *system* performance, rather than individual performance, is therefore encouraging. If such methods become more widely adopted, they may substantially alter the process of evaluating and credentialing physicians by focusing instead on the processes that help or hinder them in doing their jobs (Koska, 1991; Deming, 1986). Instead of blaming a practitioner for failing to achieve a given standard of performance, managers would ask, "Where has the system failed, and why?" Focusing on the processes of care takes the onus off of individual actors and makes it easier to establish an identity of interests around systemwide efforts to improve the quality of clinical care.

Coordination and Integration of Clinical Support Systems

Let us now consider some of the problems patients experience with ancillary systems of clinical support, and their possible solutions.

Problems

Most of the high technology of "high-technology" medicine is to be found in clinical support services—the diagnostic tests and therapeutic procedures that physicians order for their patients to support clinical decision making and clinical care. Here, especially, given the technical sophistication of the equipment and procedures, quality and effectiveness must be assessed by technical experts: Is equipment state-of-the-art, up to date, and in good working order? Are technicians well trained and competent? Are utilization and ordering patterns appropriate? Are proper procedures followed?

Patients, however, have a slightly different perspective on these services. They have tremendous respect for the technology, of course, and they expect to have access to the newest and the best. Still, it is this aspect of medical care that seems to bother them most. They complain about long waits with no one telling them what's going on; they complain about pain, discomfort, humiliation, and indignity. What do these experiences and perceptions tell us about clinical support services that monitoring according to technical standards and protocols does not?

How well is the system working? First of all, because patients experience the flow of activity relating to tests and procedures in ways that other actors in the system do not, they may be able to see functional problems or inefficiencies that others miss. If they complain about unanticipated waits, delays, or postponements, for example, what are the sources of these delays? Are there difficulties with equipment, with technicians or staffing, or with the dissemination of information?

Quality improvement experts tell us that the first question to ask in probing a problem or following up a complaint is whether the observed problem is an aberration or deviation from the norm or a regular occurrence. Answering this question may require analyzing the observations of many different patients over time, as well as gathering additional data to augment those observations—data on actual waiting times, for instance, or on the number of times tests were rescheduled. If the problem is short term or a haphazard occurrence, it probably reflects some sort of temporary system failure—an unusual increase in demand, or a breakdown in equipment, or a temporary shortage of personnel. If, on the other hand, it is a regular occurrence, the trouble most likely resides in the system, itself (Berwick, Godfrey, and Roessner, 1990; Deming, 1986). Precisely because they have become part of routine operating procedures, such difficulties may not be visible to regular actors in the system. And it is here that patients—as "outside" participant-observers who nonetheless have a critical stake in the process—can be especially astute witnesses. They may not be able to diagnose what is wrong, but they can often see the "cracks" in the system as well as the institutionalized inefficiencies.

Diagnosing a problem within an organizational system entails what systems analysts and quality consultants sometimes describe as "peeling back the onion" to uncover deeper layers of causal relationships. Berwick, Godfrey, and Roessner (1990) tell of a Japanese quality improvement expert who advises his clients to ask "why" at least five times to help them peel deeper and deeper. The *first* "why" may well come from patients.

Are patients' needs and perceptions being taken into account? The diagnostic and therapeutic procedures that patients submit to during the course of their medical treatment are often the most painful, disturbing, and dehumanizing parts of the whole experience. What may be routine to clinicians and technicians is anything but that to patients. Gilda Radner (1989, pp. 60–61), once again, has vividly described her personal experience with that relatively common diagnostic procedure, the barium enema: "The technicians strapped me to a table and then put a tube in my rear end. As they poured a chalky liquid inside me and pumped gas into me so that my bowel would show up . . . , they were also turning me slowly around and around on the table. . . . I had never had a photo session quite like this. . . . I felt like I was trapped on an endless Ferris wheel with someone's fist up my butt. . . . I think the word that best captures the whole event is *humiliating*." Much of the discomfort and physical humiliation may be unavoidable. But other patients describe what seems to be gratuitous degradation: being processed assembly-line style by technicians they do not know, who do not explain what they are doing; being manipulated like slabs of meat on cold stainless steel tables; being left half-naked in public corridors or waiting areas; being told, wrongly, that "this won't hurt."

Why is this so? Part of the problem is that for most diagnostic tests and procedures, the primary "customer" is the doctor—*not* the patient. What matters is how quickly, accurately, and completely information is conveyed to the clinician to help rule out possibilities or confirm a diagnosis. Patients (or their bodily parts) are the subjects of investigation, in this schema, whose needs and perceptions can easily be overlooked. Moreover, the technicians whose job it is to prep, draw blood, or perform tests and procedures encounter each patient only briefly—just long enough, from the patient's point of view, to poke, jab, scrape, photograph, or zap. These are hardly circumstances conducive to the establishment of a sensitive personal relationship. Perhaps for this reason, such jobs are usually defined more in terms of the technical tasks to be performed than in terms of patient care. Those who work in these positions tend to be evaluated more for their skill and efficiency in performing their assigned tasks than for their sensitivity in dealing with patients (Deming, 1986).

Do patients and their families understand what services, procedures, or consultations are to be ordered, when they are to occur, how long they will take, and what effect they might have? Much of the stress, anxiety, and frustration that patients express about medical tests and procedures has less to do with the experience itself than with the apprehension that comes from not knowing what is going to happen. "It was the waiting. The waiting drove him nuts," one wife of a cardiac patient explained, echoing a familiar sentiment in the focus group. Patients often know that critical clinical decisions hang on the outcome of certain tests, but they may have no more than a vague idea of when those tests will occur, until the escort arrives with the wheelchair or stretcher to take them there. Once there, they may well have to wait again, in a holding area, often without company or explanation.

Nor do they always know what to expect, although enough explanation will likely have been given about the more invasive, painful, or risky procedures to raise their level of anxiety. Even tests that seem relatively innocuous to the technicians administering them may be alarming to patients because of the equipment involved or the unexpected physical sensations they cause. One focus-group patient described her experience with a diagnostic imaging procedure that required the injection of a tracer dye: "She [the technician injecting the dye] said, 'You might feel a little sting or a little heat in your throat.' Well, that was the understatement of the year!

I got a retching throat! She said, 'Well, about 60 percent of the patients do that, but we don't want to tell them because it will lead to more work. It's really not serious.' " One of every five patients we surveyed nationally reported that no one told them what pain or discomfort to expect during tests and procedures. And as one patient put it, "The unknown is sometimes scarier than what they tell you." The imagination, fueled by the knowledge that something is wrong and a fear of the unknown, can conjure up images far worse than any reality.

Solutions

From the patients' point of view, good diagnostic and therapeutic support services are those that run smoothly and predictably, without obvious foul-ups or delays, while also taking into account the patients' needs and comforts. Providing such services requires recognizing patients as the clinic's "customers," and not just the subjects of its investigations. It also requires paying serious attention to what patients experience when they undergo tests and procedures.

Sometimes the brusqueness or insensitivity of laboratory technicians or other ancillary personnel masks their own sense of inadequacy in dealing with sick and frightened patients. Many of the "guest relations" and "service excellence" programs that hospitals have launched in recent years aim to help such technically trained workers understand patients' needs and redefine their own work accordingly. To be effective, however, such programs must go beyond what some workers refer to derogatorily as "smile school." They must also help redesign support systems to serve patients' needs (Crosby, 1979; Leebov, 1988; Berwick, Godfrey, and Roessner, 1990; Carlzon, 1987). Far from making "more work," as the technician in the story above apparently believed, accommodating patients' needs will actually lead to *less* work. Built into the scheduling protocols for virtually every test and procedure offered at the Mayo Clinic, for example, is the patient's age, gender, functional status, and any other known factor that might affect the person's preparation, tolerance, or recovery. And for this reason, the design and operation of clinical support services at the Mayo Clinic are truly a marvel of efficiency. In other settings, technicians may roll their eyes and sigh when they see a "difficult" patient arrive, anticipating the "delays" or headaches the person is likely to cause. But the planners at Mayo, recognizing how hard it is to design patients to fit the system, have designed a system that fits the real patients who are their customers.

At Mayo, too, patients know what to expect during the course of their stay. Within an hour after their initial examination, they will know exactly what tests have been scheduled; exactly when and where they will take place; exactly how long they will take; and exactly what they will entail. In inpatient settings, of course, such predictability may not be possible, given the unforeseeable demands on the system. Still, patients want to know as much as they can about what will happen to them, even if the plans change. It helps them regain a sense of control. One patient described, with gratitude, how his nurse "took me under her wing [and] told me what to expect by the hour the next day." Patients in New York University Hospital's Cooperative Care Unit are given daily schedules of their "appointments" with doctors, nurses, and clinics, even though the schedules have to be revised and updated frequently.

Redesigning systems to meet patients' needs may seem like a formidable task, but keeping them informed is a relatively simple and effective way to ease their anxiety. At Riverside Hospital in Columbus, Ohio, for example, signs are posted prominently in laboratory and clinic waiting areas telling patients how long they should expect to wait and asking them to tell the receptionist if they are kept waiting longer. The signs, of course, do nothing to change the reality of the waiting. Instead, they manage patients' *expectations* and give them a legitimate avenue for expressing a grievance if those expectations are not met (Levitt, 1986; Albrecht and Zemke, 1985). This simple device also provides immediate feedback to clinic personnel when the system is not working.

Coordination and Integration of the Delivery of Patient Care

In this final section, we turn our attention to the problems of coordinating patient care at the bedside and to some possible approaches to solving them.

Problems

If the organization and operation of clinical care and clinical support services are confusing and sometimes bewildering to patients, it is because they see only a part of what is going on, on the basis of which they make judgments about the whole. On the other hand, the patient's bed is the perfect vantage point for watching and observing the care that is delivered to them personally. This "frontline" care most directly affects their experience of hospital or health care, and much of their judgment about the quality of that care is based on this experience. What, then, do patients see that shapes their judgments?

Does the patient know whom to ask for help, and is the right person available at the right time? When W. Edwards Deming, the widely acknowledged "father" of quality improvement, was a hospital patient, he remarked in a memorandum (1987) on his experience how often the person who answered his call button was not able to help him. Typically, an aide or ward helper would respond to the light, tell him that his request was someone else's domain, cancel the call light, and then leave. Deming's frustration trying, in his prone and bedridden position, to track the right person down has a familiar ring to almost anyone who has ever been a hospital patient. Patients do not know whose job it is to do what, and nearly one-third (31 percent) of those we surveyed nationally were not even told who to ask when they needed help. But to ward personnel, "answering lights" (like "answering the phone" to office workers) tends to be seen as an annoying and mindless task, and it may therefore fall to the staff person with the least power to refuse. A person so chosen is not likely to have the power, authority, or knowledge to deliver patients what they want or need.

Quality consultants to service organizations emphasize the importance of empowering front-line workers to deliver services to clients, answer their questions, and solve their problems (Leebov and Scott, 1990). Albrecht and Zemke (1985, p. 85) suggest two simple measures as a "litmus test" of an organization's effectiveness in this regard: "The next time you telephone an organization, . . . count the number of interdepartmental transfers you go through before you get anything resembling help. Next, count the number of people who explain to you why they can't help you because the thing you want to know or have done is the responsibility of . . . some other unit." Substituting a patient's request for the hypothetical telephone inquiry, front-line patient care in hospital environments would often receive low marks on such a test, for several reasons.

First, as in the case Deming has described, those who come into contact with a patient at any given time may not have the authority, knowledge, or training to provide the needed service. Staff members who have not been clinically trained at a given level, for example, cannot and should not give medications or change dressings. Kitchen workers who deliver trays cannot, on their own authority, change a patient's diet if the patient asks them to do so. Housekeepers cannot move a bedridden patient. The division of tasks on the ward may also serve workers' needs to differentiate professional status or preserve prerogatives. Staff members with professional training may resent and resist performing menial tasks, and these privileges of status may be written into formal job descriptions. Lower-status workers may also want to distinguish explicitly what they will and will not do as part of their job, to defend themselves against the encroachments of higher-ups, and these distinctions, too, may be formalized and strictly enforced (Coser, 1962). And finally, job distinctions on the ward reflect practical divisions of labor that have been institutionalized, bureaucratically, into separate departments, each governed by its own rules and standards (Leebov, 1988; Berwick, Godfrey, and Roessner, 1990). Nursing personnel at all levels thus work according to the rules and practices of the nursing department, which supervises them. Housekeepers are trained by a different department, through which they report. Dietary workers report through still another structure, and laundry workers through yet another.

Whatever the rationale for this division of labor, the bedridden patient, in the course of an average day, confronts not one but many different front-line workers, each of whose ability to respond to patients' needs is limited by an invisible set of rules (Coser, 1962).

Are front-line staff well informed? The problems that Deming encountered with the ward helper who answered his call button were twofold: first, she could not personally help him, and second, she apparently did not know, except in a general way, who could. Lacking both the skills and authority to help him and the information she needed to identify someone who could, her job was simply to "turn off the call light"—just as the temporary office secretary who is told only to "answer the phone" can do little more than stop the ringing. The staff person cited in this particular story may not have been the most diligent worker in the world—we have no way of knowing. But even the most qualified and motivated people will be rendered incompetent if they do not have the information they need to do their job. Yet front-line workers in hospitals—those who have the most direct and frequent contact with patients—may be relatively uninformed for several reasons. Ironically, it may be by design (Quint, 1965). In traditional hierarchical organizations (like many hospitals), access to information is often limited by status and function—whether to preserve professional prerogatives, protect confidentiality, or prevent misinformation. Subordinates who inquire about the organization's operations, or about whose job it is to do what, may even be told, "Don't worry about that. All *you* need to know is. . . ." One hospital unit manager, acknowledging this tendency in his own institution, quipped, "We don't want anyone to know too much, you see, in case they're captured by the enemy."

Adding to this tendency in hospitals is the real need to respect patients' privacy and to preserve the confidentiality of medical information. Hospitals therefore usually restrict access to medical records and clinical information even among their own employees. In some institutions, only the physician and the nurse in charge of a patient are formally permitted to see a patient's record. As a result, many of those who come into regular contact with patients—aides, orderlies, technicians, ward helpers, transport workers, housekeepers, dietary workers—know very little about the workings of the hospital, except from the vantage point of their own jobs, and even less about the patients they see. The close control of information may not be a liability if one person (usually the doctor) is clearly in charge and accessible, and if the lines of authority and responsibility are relatively simple, clear, and recognized. Under those circumstances, both patients and staff will likely know where to turn for the help and information they need. As responsibility becomes more diffuse, however, limiting access to information can be counterproductive.

Are direct patient care functions effectively coordinated? Deming, in his capacity as hospital patient, also timed how long it took his nurse to be "back in a minute," as he lay in a state of undress waiting to get help bathing, or to have his dressing changed, or to have his bed made. It literally took hours, repeatedly. He did not blame the nurse—she was clearly very busy (Deming, 1987). Much, perhaps even most, of the care that patients find themselves in need of, as they lie in their hospital beds—help with eating, bathing, or going to the bathroom, changing bed linens, replacing water pitchers, emptying bedpans, and so forth—has little to do with clinical care per se. Such services are often defined as secondary activities of the nursing staff, and as such they are likely to be assigned a relatively low priority, given the other demands on nurses' time. Of the hospital patients we surveyed nationally, 28 percent found, like Deming, that their nurses were at times "too busy" to take care of them.

Many aspects of direct patient service—housekeeping, linen service, dietary, and so on—are also the jobs of ancillary service workers who report through separate functionally defined bureaucratic hierarchies. At the point of "service delivery" (the patient's bedside), responsibilities may be ill-defined and poorly coordinated, even though people are busy doing their jobs. Even when problems are recognized, they often remain unresolved, because no one below the level of top management has the recognized authority to settle jurisdictional disputes. Typically, such disputes are referred "up the line" through the separate reporting structures, where they compete with more urgent problems for management's attention (Leebov and Scott, 1990). Patients will probably not know, or care, that the nurses on one shift resent being stuck with the "scut" work left behind by another shift, that nurses think emptying wastebaskets is the housekeepers' job and housekeepers think it's the nurses' job, or that kitchen workers and nursing staff battle routinely over who should deliver and collect meal trays. The patients will see, though, that dressings have not been changed, wastebaskets not emptied, food trays not picked up. And given the mystery and dread that shrouds much of what else happens to them in hospitals, that may be what they see most clearly and most prominently.

Solutions

Of the three tasks of coordination discussed in this chapter, coordinating service at the bedside is probably the one that hospitals throughout the country have addressed most explicitly. The impetus has come mainly from two directions. First, from nursing: bedside care is most often identified as the domain of nursing, and nurses have been instrumental in exploring alternative methods of organizing and delivering bedside patient care. And second, from management: because it is the aspect of hospital care that patients and their families see most directly, and the one least dependent on the involvement of physicians, hospital administrators and service quality consultants have also turned their attention to the development of more patient-focused bedside care.

Nursing initiatives, although many and varied in their purpose and design, have generally relied on a two-pronged strategy designed to enhance the role of nurses and improve the quality of bedside care. Such strategies often involve some restructuring of jobs and reporting patterns, giving nurses either direct or supervisory responsibility over those aspects of patient services typically carried out by nonnursing staff. They may also entail giving nursing a larger role in hospital governance, while increasing the accountability and responsibility of the nurses on the front lines of patient care. The aim is to give a more central role in coordinating and delivering services to those who are most knowledgeable about the patients. For example, the primary nursing model—one of the most widely publicized among recent nursing innovations—assigns one experienced nurse (usually trained at the baccalaureate level or above) primary responsibility for all aspects of bedside care for a given patient throughout that patient's hospital stay. It is important to bear in mind, however, that what seems efficient and well coordinated from a nursing perspective can still be confusing and frustrating to patients. Even under the purest form of primary nursing, a patient will have at least three and perhaps as many as six different nurses during a given stay, and the designated primary nurse may not be the one most often encountered. Moreover, nurses are likely to have a different set of priorities than patients, and some subjectively important tasks can still fall through the cracks.

Borrowing from successful models in other service industries, other hospital innovators have also promoted elaborate restructuring of staffing, task assignments, and reporting structures in an effort to break down bureaucratic barriers at the point of service delivery, promote coordination, empower front-line staff, and improve patient services. One consulting group's experimental model for patient-focused care has decentralized such ancillary patient care services as admissions, radiology, pharmacy, and routine laboratory work to the unit level and has cross-trained nurses in phlebotomy, physical therapy, and respiratory therapy. The model unit has also redesigned physical space to bring supplies and services closer to the patient and has coordinated all activities through patient care "partnerships" headed by nurses (Brice, 1991). Others have experimented with variations on the themes of decentralization, cross-training, and coordination of ancillary care through nursing, in an effort to "empower" front-line workers and bring services closer to patients.

Still other hospitals have experimented with ways to improve patients' access to services within existing organizational structures. Mercy Hospital in Roseburg, Oregon, for example, employs ward clerks on each unit twenty-four hours a day and has everyone in the hospital—including all nurses, central supply clerks, and other ancillary workers—carry a beeper. The ward clerk, who is trained to know who in the hospital is responsible for what, can answer a patient's call button and contact the appropriate person directly and immediately. Patient call-light systems now commercially available also have the capacity to give patients direct access to the particular services they need, eliminating the need for an intermediary.

Our own findings from the field suggest that the success of any given nursing or managerial model will depend in large part on the culture and environment of the institution in which it is applied. There is no one model for success. Although some of the more elaborate restructuring experiments hold the promise of dramatically revolutionizing patient services, they also have to contend with some of the stiffest sources of professional and bureaucratic resistance. It is too early to know how these experiments will fare in the long run, and which structural innovations will turn out to be worth the effort.

In the meantime, improving patient care at the bedside need not entail radical changes in structure or staffing patterns. Two more modest themes recurred among the patient-centered hospitals we visited. Most obvious was the tendency to define all jobs in a hospital in terms that clearly recognize the importance of patients' perceptions and experiences. At Trinity Hospital in Minot, North Dakota, for example, housekeepers told us that their first responsibility is to clean patients' rooms, treatment areas, and public areas. In times past, administrative offices had taken top priority. Staff training at the Mayo Clinic and its affiliated hospitals similarly frames each job clearly in terms of its impact on patients. The University of Chicago Hospitals developed a "Patient-Centered Care Guidelines Worksheet" to stimulate thought and discussion among caregivers at all levels and to develop guidelines for care (Fullam, 1991). The tool is a simple matrix, listing the dimensions of patient-centered care vertically and groups of caregivers horizontally. It provides a visible structure to help all staff members think about their own contribution to patient care.

The second common theme among the more successful patient-centered hospitals we visited was a tendency among lower-level, front-line staff to take the initiative to solve their own problems, including those that involved jurisdictional disputes, instead of passing the buck onto higher levels of management. In some hospitals, staff had always functioned this way; in others, it required a conscious and deliberate effort to encourage and reward initiative. As one quality officer in a large academic health center told us, "A lot of our departmental supervisors didn't know it was okay to talk to each other. Their first inclination when a problem arose was to write a memo to their superior." Success in her hospital was measured by the decrease in the number of such memos generated. The vice president for nursing at another hospital routinely sends items that come to her desk "back down the line," telling the nurse managers to take care of the matter themselves. "Sooner or later," she says, "they get the message." One positive outcome can be seen in the practical arrangements that nursing and dietary staff have worked out for the delivery and pickup of meal trays—an ongoing dispute that had resisted resolution because of the apparently idiosyncratic needs of each unit. The solution was to have the nurses and dietary workers on each unit work out whatever arrangements suited them best.

Summary

Patients and their families are eyewitnesses to the processes of health care delivery. They will sense that they are in good, competent hands if the care they receive seems effectively coordinated, integrated into a coherent system of care, and cognizant of their individual needs and circumstances. On the other hand, care that appears uncoordinated or disintegrated, no matter how "good" it might be by some other external measure of quality, will *not* instill in patients feelings of confidence or trust. Health care institutions face three distinct coordinative tasks in the delivery of care: (1) coordination of clinical care, across specialty and professional lines; (2) coordination of clinical support and ancillary services; and (3) coordination of the various, sometimes specialized tasks that make up care at the bedside.

The coordination of clinical care is complicated by the multiplicity of players involved and the diffuse lines of authority among them. To patients, it may appear that no one is in charge—and in a literal sense, perhaps no *one* is. Patients may be left to sort out complicated information and sometimes conflicting messages on their own. Members of the clinical team need to clarify the lines of authority and responsibility—among themselves, as well as to patients. Physicians, who bear ultimate responsibility for clinical care, must also play the central, coordinating role, although members of the team who have closer or more frequent contact with patients may be appropriate conduits of information. Strategies that seek to involve physicians in efforts to improve the clinical processes of care may be more effective than those that gauge their performance according to external norms or standards.

Laboratory tests and procedures are often bewildering to the patients who undergo them, because such services are designed primarily to support clinical decision makers and only indirectly to serve patients. In the process, patients' more immediate needs and perceptions can be lost sight of. Managers need to elicit feedback from patients about the operation of such services and reexamine them with patients' needs in mind. Such feedback can also be useful in revealing operational problems that might otherwise go unnoticed. When delays, discomfort, and other causes of distress cannot be eliminated or avoided, letting patients know clearly what to expect can ameliorate their negative effects.

Patients lying in their hospital beds do not understand much about the division of labor on the ward or about job definitions or reporting structures. They are not in a position to search out what they need, although they may need help with even the most mundane aspects of daily living. The routine aspects of bedside care may be assigned to different staff members in different departments, whose work priorities may not be consonant with patients' subjective needs. Although a variety of alternative staffing models have been designed to improve the coordination of bedside care, no single model will be effective in every hospital setting. Managers must review practices within their own institutions and, in the context of their own organizational cultures, ensure that (1) patients have ready access to effective help with their subjective needs and problems, and (2) staff who come into regular contact with patients have the knowledge, authority, and explicit responsibility to solve those problems and meet those needs.

Suggestions for Improvement

- Give patients written and/or visual information identifying members of the clinical team, explaining the role of each, and identifying the clinician in charge of their care.
- Solicit patients' perceptions about the coordination of clinical care (for example, whether they understand the roles of team members; whether the information they get is consistent) and make this information available to the clinician in charge.
- Use patient feedback to solicit physicians' help in improving the coordination of care.
- Have the clinical team identify one person to serve as the primary conduit of information for the patient and family—pref-

erably a clinician regularly in contact with the patient, such as a primary nurse, resident, or attending physician.

- Ask patients regularly about their experiences with clinical tests and procedures—for instance, about waiting times, delays, pain or discomfort, and the information they were given.

- Use patient feedback to develop guidelines and explicit standards for laboratory technicians and others to follow when dealing with patients.

- Give patients and their families realistic expectations about waiting times, levels of discomfort, possible side effects, and other factors relating to tests and procedures.

- Identify factors (such as age, functional status, possible side effects) that might predictably influence a patient's tolerance of or recovery from a clinical test or procedure, and design protocols to accommodate patients' individual needs and responses.

- Assign explicit responsibility for answering call lights on the ward, and make sure that the person who has that responsibility also has the ability or the necessary information to get patients what they want or need.

- Identify and eliminate unproductive and unnecessarily rigid divisions of labor among ward personnel. Train staff to perform a variety of caring functions for patients.

- Identify and eliminate unnecessary barriers to information. Give all staff who come in regular contact with a patient information about special needs, activity restrictions, and other appropriate information. Educate all staff about hospital and ward organization, work structure, and job descriptions.

- Encourage staff at all levels to collaborate to solve problems and reward them for doing so.

References

Albrecht, K., and Zemke, R. *Service America! Doing Business in the New Economy.* Homewood, Ill.: Dow Jones–Irwin, 1985.

Berwick, D. M., Godfrey, A. B., and Roessner, J. *Curing Health Care: New Strategies for Quality Improvement.* San Francisco: Jossey-Bass, 1990.

Brice, J. "Patient-Focused Care at Bishop Clarkson Hospital Scores

Improvements in Patient Satisfaction and Worker Productivity in a Radical New Design of the Hospital Workplace." *Healthcare Productivity Report,* 1991, *4,* 1-10.

Carlzon, J. *Moments of Truth.* New York: Ballinger, 1987.

Coser, R. L. "Authority and Decision Making in a Hospital: A Comparative Analysis." *American Sociological Review,* 1958, *23,* 56-63.

Coser, R. L. *Life in the Ward.* East Lansing: Michigan State University Press, 1962.

Crosby, P. B. *Quality Is Free: The Art of Making Quality Certain.* New York: New American Library, 1979.

Deming, W. E. *Out of the Crisis.* Cambridge: Center for Advanced Engineering Study, Massachusetts Institute of Technology, 1986.

Deming, W. E. "Notes on Management in a Hospital." Unpublished memorandum, 1987.

Freidson, E. *Profession of Medicine: A Study in the Sociology of Applied Knowledge.* New York: Dodd-Mead, 1970.

Fullam, F. A. "Using a Worksheet to Help Implement Patient-Centered Care." *Picker/Commonwealth Report,* 1991, *1,* 2.

Ingelfinger, F. "Arrogance." *New England Journal of Medicine,* 1980, *303,* 1507-1511.

Inguanzo, J. M., and Harju, M. "What Makes Consumers Select a Hospital?" *Hospitals,* 1985, *59,* 90-94.

Knaus, W. A., Draper, E. A., Wagner, D. P., and Zimmerman, J. E. "An Evaluation of Outcome from Intensive Care in Major Medical Centers." *Annals of Internal Medicine,* 1986, *104,* 410-418.

Koeck, C., and Levitt, S. "Continuous Quality Improvement and the Organizational Behavior Literature." Unpublished manuscript, Harvard School of Public Health, 1990.

Koska, M. T. "Quality Improvement Methods Influence Privileging Process." *Hospitals,* July 5, 1991, p. 78.

Lebow, J. L. "Consumer Assessment of the Quality of Medical Care." *Medical Care,* 1974, *12,* 328-337.

Leebov, W. *Service Excellence: The Customer Relations Strategy for Health Care.* Chicago: American Hospital Publishing, 1988.

Leebov, W., and Scott, G. *Health Care Managers in Transition: Shifting Roles and Changing Organizations.* San Francisco: Jossey-Bass, 1990.

Levitt, T. *The Marketing Imagination*. New York: Free Press, 1986.

Lidz, C. W., and others. "Barriers to Informed Consent." *Annals of Internal Medicine*, 1983, *99*, 539-543.

McIntosh, J. "Processes of Communication, Information Seeking, and Control Associated with Cancer: A Selective Review of the Literature." *Social Science and Medicine*, 1974, *8*, 167-187.

Omachonu, V. K. "Quality of Care and the Patient: New Criteria for Evaluation." *Health Care Management Review*, 1990, *15*, 43-50.

Palmer, R. H., Strain, R., Rothrock, J. K., and Hsu, L. "Evaluation of Operational Failures in Clinical Decision Making." *Medical Decision Making*, 1983, *3*, 299-310.

Press, I. "The Predisposition to File Claims: The Patient's Perspective." *Law, Medicine, and Health Care*, 1984, *12*, 53-62.

Quint, J. C. "Institutionalized Practices of Information Control." *Psychiatry*, 1965, *28*, 119-132.

Radner, G. *It's Always Something*. New York: Avon Books, 1989.

Steiber, S. R. "How Consumers Perceive Health Care Quality." *Hospitals*, Apr. 5, 1988, p. 84.

Wadler, J. "My Breast: One Woman's Cancer Story." Part 2. *New York*, Apr. 20, 1992, pp. 48-60.

Wennberg, J. E. "Outcomes Research, Cost Containment, and the Fear of Health Care Rationing." *New England Journal of Medicine*, 1990, *323*, 1202-1204.

Wessen, A. F. "Hospital Ideology and Communication Between Ward Personnel." In E. G. Jaco (ed.), *Patients, Physicians, and Illness*. New York: Free Press, 1958.

4

Overcoming
the Barrier of Words

Jennifer Daley

"All my life I have listened to practitioners saying one thing and patients hearing another," the physician Edward E. Rosenbaum tells us in his best-selling book *The Doctor*. He recalls one especially compelling example of such miscommunication: "When I was in medical school, a bright ten-year-old girl was admitted because of diabetes. She was so uncooperative that the frustrated staff could not deal with her. In desperation, a psychologist was brought to see her. He explained the problem to the staff. The child was sure she was dying. She had heard her doctor describing her case to the students, and when she heard him say that she had diabetes, she interpreted it to mean she would 'die of beeties.' "

We live in the golden age of communication—telecommunications, informatics, computer networking, conference calls, the global village, "on-the-spot" reporting, overnight mail, and fax technology. At times, it seems we are inundated with more factual information and communications than we can hope to assimilate, understand, and process. In the hospital, most of the administrative, clinical, and interpersonal activities are devoted to communication. Simply reflecting on the ever-increasing amount of mail (electronic or otherwise), telephone calls, "faxes," laboratory reporting and computer systems, telecommunication networks and linkages, meetings, case conferences, newsletters, bulletins, memorandums, and

72

junk mail generated every day in most hospitals can be overwhelming. These systems are built to make the process of caring for patients both more effective and more efficient. In their conceptualization, these modes of communication are intended to provide more information in a timely and efficient way to facilitate caring for patients. And yet in the midst of instantaneous transmission of clinical information and constant striving for more efficiency, it seems that more information is transferred but less is communicated. Patients and their human experience of illness and health are lost or overlooked.

Communication is defined as the transmission of information, thoughts, and feelings so that they are satisfactorily received or understood. In some sense, this entire book is about communication *through the patient's eyes.* Prior and subsequent chapters discuss in detail patients' and their families' experience in describing their pain and suffering to medical professionals and, in response, receiving care that addresses both the technical and the nontechnical aspects of caring. We discuss important aspects of pain management, emotional support, patient education, respect for patient preferences, the transition out of hospital, and the family's role and needs during hospitalization. Each of these dimensions involves communication as a critical and necessary ingredient in patient-centered care. In this chapter, we begin to discuss—from the patients' perspective—some of the issues in communication that may arise between patients and their caregivers, physicians and nurses. We will describe some general interventions that have proved innovative and helpful in facilitating communication; many of these interventions and suggestions for improvement are elaborated on in subsequent chapters.

Communication: Is It Important?

Communication of information, thoughts, and feelings is critical to both the technical and nontechnical aspects of caring for patients. In the technical aspects of care, active exchange of information is critical to establishing diagnosis and treatment. Most of the information essential to the technical success of medical care is elicited by providers from patients. Patients relate their symptoms and concerns; providers review these symptoms in the context of their prior experience and knowledge and ask for more information from the patients and additional data from physical and laboratory examination. Indeed, the success or failure of arriving at the correct diagnosis and appropriate therapy is predicated on effective exchange of information. Providers are then responsible for communicating to the patients their opinion about the nature of the problem, what action should be taken to correct the problem, and the likelihood that the problem can be alleviated, as well as for determining that the patients have understood and agree with the course of action outlined.

By definition, communication about the technical aspects of care is lopsided. The patient possesses the full richness of the experience of illness but little in the way of expert knowledge about what this experience means in the scientific biomedical construct. The provider abstracts or distills the patient's experience into one of several known biomedical explanations and prepares to intervene and reassure the patient. Regarding the technical aspects of care, the patient is less knowledgeable, more passive, and more vulnerable than the provider.

In the patient-centered aspects of care, communication between the patient and the provider is equally important but critically different. Through the patient's eyes, communication is the essential ingredient to participation in healing and recovery. As one of the patients we spoke with said, "information is my food." In this realm, however, the communication is not restricted to facts, diagnoses, recommended treatments, and likelihoods of recovery. Greater emphasis is placed on expressing deep feelings and subjective experience. Nonverbal forms of communication such as touching, listening, gesturing, posturing, facial expression, and tone express the human condition of health and illness. In this aspect of caring, the patient and the provider are on equal ground. Neither is a novice or an expert in communicating feeling. The communication between them is more mutual (Carter, Inui, Kukull, and Haigh, 1982; Wasserman and Inui, 1983).

Communication in the technical aspects of medical care is acknowledged to be essential. We cannot make appropriate diagnoses and work with patients to treat their illness without communication. Can patients and their caregivers do without patient-centered communication? We assert throughout this book that neither patients nor their caregivers can fully experience healing and recovery from illness in the absence of communication in the patient-centered realms of care. From Plato in classical times (Inui and Carter, 1985) to Peabody in the 1920s (1927) to modern medical sociologists such as Waitzkin (Waitzkin and Stoeckle, 1976; Waitzkin, 1984; Suchman and Matthews, 1988), patients and caregivers have described more healing in patients and greater satisfaction in caregivers when patient-centered care is central to both.

Does this really matter in helping patients through their illness experience? Do patients actually have better outcomes when the communication between them and their caregivers improves? Several studies suggest that improved communication has a significant impact on patient satisfaction. Roter and others (Roter, Hall, and Katz, 1987) noted a positive impact on patient satisfaction, recall of medical advice, and overall impression of outpatient visits if the physician consistently used patient-centered skills such as giving information and counseling, rather than physician-centered behaviors such as giving directions and asking questions.

In a related study of return visits by over 500 medical outpatients (Bertakis, Roter, and Putnam, 1991), several significant relationships between communication during the visit and patient satisfaction were identified through detailed analysis of physician-patient interactions. Both physicians' questioning about biomedical topics *and* patients' talking about biomedical topics were correlated with decreased patient satisfaction. Conversely, physicians' questioning and counseling about psychosocial issues and patients' talking about these issues were all correlated with improved patient satisfaction. Patients were less satisfied when physicians dominated the interview by talking more or when the emotional tone was characterized by physician dominance. Patient satisfaction was enhanced by communication in which they were encouraged to talk about psychosocial issues in an atmosphere lacking in physician domination. A detailed analysis (Rowland-Morin and Carroll, 1990) of the language used by physicians in their initial interviews with patients suggests that three aspects of the physician's use of language—the use of silence or long reaction times between speakers in the interview, the use of the patient's own words and language by the physician, and the use of interruptions to reflect on the communication between the physician and the patient—all contributed significantly to patient satisfaction with the visit.

Improved patient-physician communication also has a positive impact on the health outcomes of patients. Kaplan, Greenfield, and others (Greenfield, Kaplan, and Ware, 1985; Greenfield and others, 1988; Kaplan, Greenfield, and Ware, 1989) demonstrated the positive impact of improving patient-physician interaction on the outcomes of chronic illness. Patients with diabetes and hypertension were educated in more effective methods of communicating their concerns to the physicians. Follow-up demonstrated that the patients who received such training had significant differences in lowering of blood sugar and blood pressure and improved quality of life.

Studies conducted in a variety of practice settings among chronically ill patients of differing sociodemographic characteristics demonstrated an improvement not only in health status measured by physiological measures, but also in functional status and overall self-reported health status. Similarly, Woolley, Kane, Hughes, and Wright (1978) studied 1,761 primary care encounters and demonstrated a relationship between both patient satisfaction and health status with communication between patient and doctor that the patient characterized as positive.

Communication: Can We Improve It?

Are we having problems communicating with our patients? Some evidence suggests that we are. In the Picker/Commonwealth survey of patients discharged from adult medical-surgical services of acute care hospitals, patients reported the most significant problems in obtaining information and communicating with their doctors and nurses in several areas. The biggest problems of clinical significance related to setting appropriate expectations about pain and discomfort during the hospitalization. Twenty-one percent of patients reported that the nurse or doctor did not explain how much discomfort to expect during a test. Nearly a quarter of all patients having surgery said that their surgeon did not explain how much discomfort they would have postoperatively and that they were not accurately informed of how they would feel after surgery. Older patients undergoing surgery and medical and surgical patients who reported their own health status as fair or poor reported receiving less information in virtually all areas. Patients cared for in public academic health centers and those without health insurance coverage reported the highest rates of difficulty in communication, although the differences were often not large. Approximately 10 percent of all patients responded that information they needed was not communicated to them; one-third of these patients wanted more information about finances and insurance.

A surprising number of anecdotal reports also suggest that we can improve our communication with patients. From the popular press to the most distinguished medical journals, observers and participants in caring for patients speak of the gulf between the technical successes of modern medicine and the growing human distance between patients and providers. Increasingly, patients feel alienated from their caregivers and complain that they "can't get any answers" and that "doctors are playing God."

In this age of consumerism, patient education specialists report that, despite advances in other areas of consumer activism, little has changed in the way patients and providers communicate. Traditional models of the authoritative physician and the passive, receptive patient who "complies" with medical recommendations still dominate the medical enterprise. Scharf (1988) reviewed twenty-five years of popular periodicals and recent self-help literature and noted numerous problems in patient-physician communication. The popular literature shows that patients perceive physicians as concealing information about diagnosis and treatment on a paternalistic basis. That is, they believe that on the pretext of trying to "protect" them, physicians withhold relevant information about their care (Lipkin, 1979; Katz, 1984; Bell, 1986).

Complaining about increasing demands on their time by third-party insurers for documentation and regulatory requirements, some physicians lament "the good old days" when patients dutifully complied with their care plans and did not ask questions about side effects of medications or risks associated with a surgical or diagnostic procedure. Some physicians express impatience with the empathic listening and communication necessary to patient-centered care, dismissing this aspect of care as too "touchy-feely." The book *The Doctor* dramatizes the story of a physician who has been diagnosed with cancer and who experiences some of the impersonal and distancing impacts of care in the hospital in which he works. His interpretation of being a patient changes as he is forced to confront the human costs of technically competent but impersonal care and experiences the emotional impact of his own illness.

Physicians themselves perceive difficulties with patient communication. A study of physicians in Great Britain by Pendleton (1983) notes that physicians feel they are ineffective as communicators in one-quarter of all their interactions with patients. Gorlin and Zucker (1983) claim that one of the roots of the failure of modern medicine is the lack of emphasis on understanding and acceptance of the physician's feelings in the patient-physician relationship.

The late Norman Cousins (1982, p. 587), in a commencement address to the George Washington University Medical School in 1982, spoke about "the physician as communicator" and the "biochemistry of the emotions." He observed that every patient comes to the physician with two diseases; the first is the disease that is diagnosed and treated and the second is panic. He noted, "I pray that when he goes into a patient's room, the physician will recognize that the main distance is not from the door to the bed but from the patient's eyes to his own and the shortest distance between those two points is a horizontal straight line—the kind of straight line that works best when the physician bends low to the patient's loneliness, fear, and pain and the overwhelming sense of mortality that comes flooding up out of the unknown, and when the physician's hand on the patient's shoulder or arm is a shelter against darkness" (p. 589).

Research on patient-provider communication has confirmed many of these perceptions. Surprisingly little of this research, however, has focused on what transpires between patients and their caregivers in the acute care hospital. Areas that have been explored include communication between physicians and patients around patient preferences for life-sustaining therapy near the end of life—such as the use of cardiopulmonary resuscitation (Bedell and Delbanco, 1984; Kohn and Menon, 1988; Frankl, Oye, and Bellamy, 1989; Schonwetter and others, 1991). Other areas that have been studied include communication of "bad news" to patients and their families (Viswanathan, Clark, and Viswanathan, 1986; Knox and Thomson, 1989; Quill and Townsend, 1991) and communication about cancer diagnosis and therapy (Klenow and Youngs, 1987; Schain, 1990; Goldberg, Guadagnoli, Silliman, and Glicksman, 1990; Seale, 1991). Communication to families about the care of severely defective or disabled children has also been explored (McKay and Hensey, 1990). Other studies have addressed communication by anesthesiologists and surgeons in the preoperative period (Richards and McDonald, 1985; Wisiak, Kroll, and List, 1991).

Most of the research has been conducted either in physician offices or the outpatient services of general hospitals. Korsch, Gozzi, and Francis (1968) studied 800 patient visits to the walk-in clinic at Children's Hospital in Los Angeles. Parents and children were studied by means of videotape of the patient-physician interactions and follow-up interview with the parents. Although 76 percent of the patients reported satisfaction by the patient's parent, 24 percent indicated dissatisfaction. Communication barriers noted between the pediatrician and mother included a lack of warmth or friendliness on the part of the doctor, failure by the doctor to take into account the patient's concerns and expectations, lack of clear explanation about the diagnosis and cause of the illness, and the use of medical jargon. Patients with higher education were more apt to express their fears and hopes to the physician and therefore had a better chance of having them responded to.

Notable in this study was that satisfactory patient-physician interaction in this walk-in setting could be achieved in short periods of time—as little as five minutes. Ineffective communication and inefficient use of time were noted on the videotapes when the physician spoke at great length without eliciting the patient's ideas and expectations, when the physician argued with the patient about language the patient used, and when the physician used repetition to try to communicate information to achieve understanding, rather than using another approach when the patient did not seem to understand.

In a follow-up study on the same group of patients, Francis,

Korsch, and Morris (1969) examined the relationship between the patients' satisfaction with the interaction between them and the physician and subsequent compliance with the prescribed regimen. Of the 800 study patients, 38 percent were moderately compliant and 11 percent were noncompliant. Key factors in noncompliance were the extent to which patients' expectations from the visit were not met, lack of warmth in the physician, and failure to receive an explanation of the diagnosis and cause of the child's illness. The complexity of the medical regimen, the seriousness of the illness as perceived by the parent, and patient satisfaction all correlated with compliance. The generalizability of these studies may be limited by the short-term, acute illnesses and episodic interactions of a pediatric walk-in clinic, but they are suggestive of problems in patient-provider interactions.

Improving Communicating with Patients: What We Learned

One of the striking observations from reviewing the popular and scientific literature on communication between patients and their caregivers is how oriented toward the physician-patient relationship and how physician oriented the observations are (Roter, Hall, and Katz, 1988; Hall, Roter, and Katz, 1988). Relatively little has been written about patients' human experience of hospitalization and the impact of the quality of communication in the hospital on the patient. The literature often focuses on the technique and skills required in the medical interview and less on the skills and interpersonal processes that contribute to the patient's experience (Anderson and Sharpe, 1991). Likewise, relatively little is written about the impact of communication between other health professionals, such as nurses and medical therapists, and patients. A good deal is known and written about communication between patients and other health professionals such as psychiatrists, psychologists, and social workers, but little is directed toward the acutely ill patient in the hospital.

What follows is a summary of what we have learned from reading the popular and medical literature, what we have heard from patients we have interviewed, and what we observed in visiting exemplary programs around the country. Many of these general observations are expanded on in subsequent chapters with more in-depth description of programs and interventions that address these patient concerns. As with all generalizations, there are exceptions and caveats; we found, however, that these themes emerged repeatedly as we met with patients and visited programs with an emphasis on patient-centered care.

In general, hospitalized patients seek more information about their condition and care than they are provided, particularly about pain and discomfort. Patients have come to expect information about their medications, plans for diagnostic and therapeutic procedures and surgery, and the indications and potential side effects of invasive and noninvasive therapies. Patients report receiving much of this information. But in the areas of pain, discomfort and expectations about discomfort, and energy levels after surgery, anesthesia, and medical illness, some patients feel they are not adequately informed of what they can expect. Patients report this most consistently about discomfort during diagnostic tests and what to expect after surgery in both the preoperative and postdischarge periods.

Hospitalized patients' needs for information and style of communication change over the course of hospitalization. Acute hospitalization represents an enormous physical and psychological stress on patients. Most patients, regardless of their stated needs for control and involvement prior to hospitalization, regress under the stress of hospitalization and under the influence of the unfamiliar culture in the hospital. Patients' physical discomfort, emotional vulnerability, illness, and prehospitalization expectations about communication all contribute to widely differing needs during the initial phase of hospitalization, which may include either diagnostic testing, acute medical therapy, or surgery. In the period after surgery or intensive medical therapy, patients' needs may change again as acute recuperation begins. Gradual changes may occur until the transition out of the hospital is anticipated and discussed. This is a period of acute stress for both the patient and family, as transfer of care from the holding environment of the hospital to home or other supportive facility is planned for. Finally, the post-hospitalization period is a time of gradual healing and reintegration of the patient, another time when needs for information and communication are intense and stressful. A specific source of stress during this time is that the mode of communication between the patient and caregivers changes dramatically. Rather than waiting for the nurse or doctor to arrive on rounds or being available immediately—as was the case in the hospital—help, advice, and support must now be obtained by telephone or home or office visit.

Hospitalized patients' needs for information change with their illness and the acuity of their clinical condition. This is an area in which it is nearly impossible to generalize. Many patients reminded us that not all patients with diabetes or asthma or AIDS or gallstones have the same needs for information and communication during hospitalization. Likewise, a patient with cancer or AIDS may have different needs for communication at different stages of the illness. Abrams (1966) noted that many cancer patients in the initial stages of diagnosis and treatment have direct and truthful communication with their physicians in an open and free manner characterized by balance and equilibrium. In the advancing stages of cancer, in which the disease has progressed or not been arrested by therapy, patients change both what they want to know and whom they ask. They may speak more freely with friends, family, and allied health personnel but rarely confront their physicians for information. In the terminal stages, some patients retreat into silence and communication may become predominantly nonverbal through physical presence, touching, and other nonverbal means of support.

Hospitalized patients' needs for information vary with individual differences. Factors that influence these differences include their age, gender, cultural background, and socioeconomic and perceived health status. Elsewhere in this volume, we discuss the variability among patients in their needs for control, expression of personal preferences in their care, and overall involvement in their care. Variability in patients' needs for information also occurs with these factors. Older patients express less need for information than younger patients. Older female patients, patients of lower socioeconomic status, and patients with poorer perceived health express less need for information and also report receiving less information in the hospital.

*How much information is actually communicated to pa-
tients varies with the patient's age, sociodemographic characteristics, income, health status, and cultural background.* Patients at risk
for ineffective communication include patients of lower socioeconomic status as measured by occupation, insurance coverage, or
income (Epstein, Taylor, and Seage, 1985; Ventres and Gordon,
1990), older patients, especially older women (Root, 1987; Weisman,
1987), and patients with poorer self-reported health status. Patients
of a different cultural, ethnic, and socioeconomic background from
their physicians are also less likely to receive information from their
doctors.

*Providers elicit relatively little about patients' preferences,
goals, and values.* Patients expect and want their values and priorities to be discussed with their physicians and nurses, but they rarely
initiate these conversations. We have addressed this issue in some
detail in Chapter Two. Patients expect to discuss their preferences
with their caregivers but expect the physician or nurse to take the
initiative in these discussions.

*Patients need time to hear, assimilate, and process informa-
tion they are given.* Patients often feel that physicians and nurses
do not give them enough time to absorb and process information.
Repetition, clarification, and dialogue about areas of confusion in
communication are helpful. A useful rule of thumb is that patients
(or any adult learner) can assimilate two or at most three critically
important pieces of information in a short time—for example, in
a twenty-minute office visit. Information or communication laden
with fear, stress, or anxiety will take longer to assimilate. It is useful, for example, to meet with patients a second time to discuss bad
or good news and begin the second meeting by asking them what
they remember of the prior meeting and any questions they have
that have arisen in the meantime. Patients want the opportunity to
discuss what has previously been discussed, but they often feel they
are not given the chance.

*Patients receive information from many different sources—
physicians, nurses, social workers, dieticians, family members,
friends, self-help groups, alternative health care providers, and the
print and visual media.* Patients, however, may withhold information provided by other sources from nurses and physicians. For

example, some patients see a variety of alternative caregivers but rarely communicate questions or suggestions from these sources to their physicians and nurses. Patients report that they feel that their doctor or nurse would not be interested in what they know, learn, or do as a result of these other visits. Both patients and physicians have told us that physicians do not appreciate the extent to which patients use other sources of information.

Patients have differing expectations of communication about both factual information and feelings and emotions from their physicians and nurses. Among those with high expectations, patients tend not to initiate dialogue about their feelings and emotional life but rather wait for the health care providers to begin discussions about emotions. They expect physicians and nurses to open channels of communication about emotions and feelings, so that they can receive validation, clarification, and support for what they are feeling.

Patients constantly compare information they receive from one person or source with information from other sources. One of the patients we interviewed told us, "I just kept asking the same question of all my doctors and nurses until I got the answer I wanted to hear." Dissonance in the information provided by different people may create fear, anxiety, misunderstanding, and anger in patients. Although all the information they receive cannot be totally consistent, it is helpful to clarify what patients know or understand from others, so that important facts or feelings can be elicited and clarified.

Patients learn by trial and error who they can trust to have valid and accurate information that is relevant to their individual circumstances. We are often reminded by patients that they are always testing to determine what "feels right" to them and their own illness experience. One patient spoke of her experience after a mastectomy: "I quickly learned what my surgeon knew something about and what he didn't. The nurses were much more helpful in teaching me about prostheses and what I needed to do to be fitted, so I just stopped asking my surgeon."

Patients are sensitive to communication among members of the health care team. Patients are acutely aware of the communications systems within hospitals, both formal and informal. They perceive their chart as a source of communication and information but see themselves as prevented from having access to the chart. They are also aware of conferences, rounds, and conversations about them and their care. They report being sensitive to what happens during patient care rounds in and around their rooms. They also are keenly aware of commitments made to them by providers and expect something to happen as a result. They are sensitive to the amount of consonance or dissonance in the messages they receive from different providers on their "team." Many patients expect that all the members of their "team" will be communicating with each other and have similar information to give them. Patients also perceive the "team" broadly to include housekeepers, transport workers, and laboratory and radiology technicians.

When different information is conveyed to patients and the facts are in conflict, they experience considerable stress, which may manifest itself as confusion, distrust, anger, or anxiety. Patients need an environment in which they can air these feelings of confusion, mistrust, or anxiety and resolve those conflicts. One of the barriers to resolution of these feelings include the patients' fear of alienating an important member of the group of professionals caring for them.

Patients have differing capacities to understand, accept, and deal with uncertainty. The communication of levels of risk and patient understanding of the concept of risk vary from patient to patient. In addition, levels of risk mean different things to patients and providers. Great potential for miscommunication exists if the patient perceives a 5 percent risk of dying as an unlikely possibility and the physician perceives the same likelihood as unacceptable. Considerable research is being conducted by Pauker, Kassirer, and others to assist in quantifying patients' and providers' perceptions of risk (Kassirer, Moskowitz, Lau, and Pauker, 1987), although much of the research is not yet accessible to the typical patient and practitioner.

Patients speak a different language from providers. Patients use "everyday" language rather than medical language, although their language changes in the hospital toward medical language. Physicians tend to speak in medical language; nurses tend to speak a mix of everyday and medical language with patients and hence often bridge the potential language gap between physicians and patients. Nurses, in this role, function as the "communication broker" between physicians and patients (Bourhis, Roth, and Mac-Queen, 1989).

Patients' literacy levels, cultural preferences, and value systems are not typically explored or understood by health care personnel. As a result, health care providers often assume that patients have the same degree of literacy, cultural likes and dislikes, and values as the prevailing hospital patient population or culture. We have already expanded on this theme in some detail in Chapter Two.

Barriers to Effective Communication

From the patients' perspective, communication with their health care providers can be improved. Yet we must acknowledge that most health care professionals are not intentionally limiting effective communication with their patients. Most health care professionals we speak with tell us that they are more than willing to improve their communication with patients. In fact, they are eager to make the experience of hospitalization more humane and caring for their patients. Many physicians tell us that they crave the inner gratification of helping others to heal not only their disease, but also their fear. We often hear, "After all, that's what I went to medical school for!" Similarly, nurses tell us that they also seek the satisfaction of caring for their patients in a way that meets their emotional and physical needs for healing and recovery.

At the same time, however, health professionals tell us of the barriers they experience in providing patient-centered care. The barrier most often cited is what they perceive as a lack of time to be with patients. Physicians and nurses note the direct and indirect pressure they feel to see more patients, to be more "productive," and to be more "cost-effective." The impact of spiraling health costs, management of clinical care by third-party and facility policies, and the perceived pressure to "keep up" with new technologies, medical knowledge, and changing regulatory requirements drains valuable energy and time away from spending time with patients.

Providers recognize that patient-centered care takes time, although often not as much as they imagine. Many physicians in the primary care practice of medicine feel, with some justification, that time spent talking with patients about psychosocial issues is devalued by others in the medical profession and the society at large. They see this reflected in the considerably higher fees given to their colleagues in more technically oriented specialties. Some physicians and nurses who have attended conferences and training sessions offered by the Picker/Commonwealth Patient-Centered Care Program seem eager to adopt new ways of communicating with patients, though many conference participants pleaded, "Teach me how to do this quickly." Patients, on the other hand, need time to express their needs for information. One study of rehabilitation patients suggested that patients needed a minimum of a twenty-minute visit for their attitudes about desiring information and participating in decision making to influence their information-seeking communication behavior (Beisecker and Beisecker, 1990).

Some health professionals also express skepticism and, at times, outright cynicism about the value of patient-centered care to the patients and institutions in which they work. They are quick to cite common examples of the differences in economic rewards between physicians and nurses who work in fields in which patient-centered care is critically important and those that require high levels of technical skill but little in the way of patient-centered skills.

What is most striking is the frequency with which health care professionals who value patient-centered care report themselves feeling devalued by some portions of society, the institutions in which they work, and even patients themselves. They describe beginning with a deeply felt commitment to patient-centered care that gradually is eroded by the environment around them. Physicians and nurses who work in exemplary institutions describe a different kind of institutional culture in which they are valued as human beings who care for others from a patient-centered perspective. "Burnout," a feeling of depletion, weariness, and emotional fatigue from giving and caring, seems to be much less prevalent in institutions that support and value their caregivers. Many of the exemplary institutions we visited had organizations that included caring as a primary foundation of the mission of the hospital. In some hospitals, a religious or cultural heritage formed the basis of patient-centeredness; in others, a charismatic individual leading the organization formed the visible source of validating and modeling patient-centered care.

As we discussed earlier, physician dominance of the patient-physician relationship is a barrier to effective communication. Despite increasing emphasis on teaching interviewing skills in medical schools and in training programs, considerable improvement can be made in teaching and reinforcing good communication and interviewing skills to physicians. Emphasis has been placed on teaching these skills early in the training of physicians, but some research indicates that, if not repeatedly practiced and reinforced, these skills recede over time. Physicians at every level need reinforcement and additional skills training in communication. The Collaborative Study Group of the Society for General Internal Medicine Task Force on the Doctor and the Patient—an outgrowth of academic general internists' interest in learning and teaching communication skills—has continued a successful effort to train and support physicians in acquiring and teaching patient communication skills (Putnam, Stiles, Jacob, and James, 1988; Quill, 1989). Other similar programs (Evans and others, 1987) have shown that patients were significantly more satisfied with physicians who had training programs in both the emotional and cognitive domains of communication. Patients reported less anxiety and more positive feelings after seeing physicians who had been in the training programs.

Just as physician dominance is a destructive barrier to satisfactory communication, patient passivity and lack of initiative are also a barrier. Educational programs and training in assertiveness for patients are helpful in bridging this barrier (Scharf, 1988). Patient education programs are discussed in Chapter Five of this book. Programs and guides that encourage patients to communicate with their physicians and nurses in writing (Thompson, Nanni, and Schwankovsky, 1990) or through tape recordings (Johnson and Adelstein, 1991) can be effective in communicating concerns, questions, and fears to caregivers. Patients who are told that their physicians encourage the asking of questions feel more in control, pose more questions, and feel more satisfied with the visit.

Summary

In health care no less than other aspects of life, we live in an era when technology can give us almost immediate access to overwhelming amounts of information. But communication entails more than access to information. It entails the transmission of information, thoughts, and feelings, such that they are satisfactorily received and understood. Few health care providers would argue with the assertion that successful communication is critical to the technical aspects of patient care. Studies also suggest that improved patient-provider communication on the nontechnical, patient-centered aspects of care has a significant impact on patient satisfaction and a positive effect on health outcomes. Nevertheless, the traditional model of the authoritative physician and the passive, receptive patient who "complies" with medical recommendations still tends to dominate the encounter.

Our explorations of the patient's perspective on communication suggest that patients, in general, seek more information than they get, although individual needs vary significantly with age, gender, and other socioeconomic factors. Informational needs also change over the course of an illness and as a function of the patient's perceived health status. Patients need time to hear, assimilate, and process the information they are given. They also want to talk about their individual goals and preferences, although few providers initiate such discussions. Patients receive information from many different sources, compare it, and learn by trial and error whom they can trust for accurate information that is relevant to their circumstances.

However gratifying it is for doctors and other caregivers to help heal not only the disease but also the fear and apprehension that go along with illness, they often perceive that they lack the time to deliver such patient-centered care. Others feel that such care is devalued—by society, by the institutions in which they work, and even by patients themselves. Both physicians and patients, too, need to learn effective communication skills, to overcome the barrier of the dominant doctor–passive patient mode of interaction.

Suggestions for Improvement

- Initiate a patient contracting program to clarify patient and provider goals.
- Try using open medical records with patients.
- Conduct regular workshops for staff physicians and house staff on improving communication with patients. Use videotapes of actual patient discussions with physicians and nurses to initiate workshops. Ask patients to comment on the quality of communication.
- Invite families and patients to write their goals for treatment in the record.
- Conduct patient educational programs in negotiation strategies for empowering patients to discuss issues with their doctors and nurses. Incorporate assertiveness training principles into these patient education programs.
- Develop and use videotapes of patients talking about their concerns during hospitalization and use them during new employee orientations and focus groups for hospital employees.
- Institute hospitalwide guest relations programs that emphasize to all employees who work with patients the patient-centered care concept.
- Provide supportive, nonjudgmental leadership from clinical staff to encourage staff physicians, nurses, and trainees in the use of videotape and focus-group feedback from patients on their experience in the hospital.
- Focus on the transition out of the hospital as a critical opportunity to improve communication. Make explicit arrangements with patients going home on how to reach health care professionals after discharge to ask questions and get help. Establish a hot line for patients to call in the week after discharge.
- Put a bulletin board beside each patient's bed and encourage the patient and family to write down their questions and concerns. Review these with the patient's physician and nurse daily.
- Conduct regularly scheduled focus groups with recently dis-

charged patients and discuss issues of communication. Tape record or videotape these group discussions and review with staff involved with the patients' care.

- Investigate and summarize the typical communication needs and patterns of the sociodemographic and cultural groups seen in your hospital. Use these to educate hospital staff. Avoid using these to stereotype patients; instead, use them to heighten staff awareness of the differences among patients.
- Identify staff members who have particular skill in translating "technical" language into "everyday" language to observe patient rounds occasionally. Encourage them to point out how to translate "technical" into "everyday" language.
- Tape record important conversations with patients and give them a copy of the tape for them to listen to again with their families. Encourage them to return with questions or confusion they had after listening to the tapes.

References

Abrams, R. D. "The Patient with Cancer—His Changing Pattern of Communication." *New England Journal of Medicine,* 1966, *274,* 317–322.

Anderson, L. A., and Sharpe, P. A. "Improving Patient and Provider Communications: A Synthesis and Review of Communication Interventions." *Patient Education and Counseling,* 1991, *17,* 99–134.

Bedell, S. E., and Delbanco, T. L. "Choices About Cardiopulmonary Resuscitation in the Hospital: When Do Physicians Talk with Patients?" *New England Journal of Medicine,* 1984, *310,* 1089–1093.

Beisecker, A. E., and Beisecker, T. D. "Patient Information-Seeking Behavior When Communicating with Doctors." *Medical Care,* 1990, *28,* 19–28.

Bell, J. N. "How Much Should Your Doctor Tell You?" *Today's Health,* July 1986, pp. 18–24.

Bertakis, K. D., Roter, D. L., and Putnam, S. M. "The Relationship of Physician Medical Interview Style to Patient Satisfaction." *Journal of Family Practice,* 1991, *32,* 175–181.

Bourhis, R. Y., Roth, S., and MacQueen, G. "Communication in the Hospital Setting: A Survey of Medical and Everyday Language Use Amongst Patients, Nurses, and Doctors." *Social Science and Medicine*, 1989, *28*, 339-346.

Carter, W. B., Inui, T. S., Kukull, W. A., and Haigh, V. H. "Outcome-Based Doctor-Patient Interaction Analysis. 2: Identifying Effective Provider and Patient Behavior." *Medical Care*, 1982, *20*, 550-566.

Cousins, N. "The Physician as Communicator." *Journal of the American Medical Association*, 1982, *248*, 587-589.

Epstein, A. M., Taylor, W. C., and Seage, G. R. "Effects of Patients' Socioeconomic Status and Physician's Training and Practice on Patient-Doctor Communication." *American Journal of Medicine*, 1985, *78*, 101-106.

Evans, B. J., and others. "A Communication Skills Programme for Increasing Patients' Satisfaction with General Medicine Consultations." *British Journal of Medical Psychology*, 1987, *60*, 373-378.

Francis, V., Korsch, B. M., and Morris, M. J. "Gaps in Doctor-Patient Communication: Patients' Response to Medical Advice." *New England Journal of Medicine*, 1969, *280*, 535-540.

Frankl, D., Oye, R. K., and Bellamy, P. E. "Attitudes of Hospitalized Patients Toward Life Support: A Survey of 200 Medical Inpatients." *American Journal of Medicine*, 1989, *86*, 645-648.

Goldberg, R., Guadagnoli, E., Silliman, R. A., and Glicksman, A. "Cancer Patients' Concerns: Congruence Between Patients and Primary Care Physicians." *Journal of Cancer Education*, 1990, *5*, 193-199.

Gorlin, R., and Zucker, H. D. "Physicians' Reactions to Patients: A Key to Teaching Humanistic Medicine." *New England Journal of Medicine*, 1983, *308*, 1059-1063.

Greenfield, S., Kaplan, S. H., and Ware, J. E., Jr. "Expanding Patient Involvement in Care: Effects on Patient Outcome." *Annals of Internal Medicine*, 1985, *102*, 520-528.

Greenfield, S., and others. "Patients' Participation in Medical Care: Effects on Blood Sugar Control and Quality of Life in Diabetes." *Journal of General Internal Medicine*, 1988, *3*, 448-457.

Hall, J. A., Roter, D. L., and Katz, N. R. "Meta-Analysis of Correlates of Provider Behavior in Medical Encounters." *Medical Care,* 1988, *26,* 657–675.

Inui, T. S., and Carter, W. B. "Problems and Prospects for Health Services Research on Provider-Patient Communication." *Medical Care,* 1985, *23,* 521–538.

Johnson, I. A., and Adelstein, D. J. "The Use of Recorded Interviews to Enhance Physician-Patient Communication." *Journal of Cancer Education,* 1991, *6,* 99–102.

Kaplan, S. H., Greenfield, S., and Ware, J. E., Jr. "Assessing the Effects of Physician-Patient Interaction on the Outcomes of Chronic Disease." *Medical Care,* 1989, *27,* S110–S127.

Kassirer, J. P., Moskowitz, A. J., Lau, J., and Pauker, S. G. "Decision Analysis: A Progress Report." *Annals of Internal Medicine,* 1987, *106,* 275–291.

Katz, J. *The Silent World of Doctor and Patient.* New York: Free Press, 1984.

Klenow, D. J., and Youngs, G. A., Jr. "Changes in Doctor/Patient Communication of a Terminal Prognosis: A Selective Review and Critique." *Death Studies,* 1987, *11,* 263–277.

Knox, J. D., and Thomson, G. M. "Breaking Bad News: Medical Undergraduate Communication Skills Teaching and Learning." *Medical Education,* 1989, *23,* 258–261.

Kohn, M., and Menon, G. "Life Prolongation: Views of Elderly Outpatients and Health Care Professionals." *Journal of the American Geriatrics Society,* 1988, *36,* 840–844.

Korsch, B. M., Gozzi, E. K., and Francis, V. "Gaps in Doctor-Patient Communication. 1: Doctor-Patient Interaction and Patient Satisfaction." *Pediatrics,* 1968, *42,* 855–871.

Lipkin, M. "On Lying to Patients." *Newsweek,* June 4, 1979, p. 13.

McKay, M., and Hensey, O. "From the Other Side: Parents' View of Their Early Contacts with Health Professionals." *Child: Care, Health, and Development,* 1990, *16,* 373–381.

Peabody, F. W. "The Care of the Patient." *Journal of the American Medical Association,* 1927, *88,* 877–882.

Pendleton, D. "Doctor-Patient Communication: A Review." in D. Pendleton and J. Hasler (eds.), *Doctor-Patient Communication.* London: Academic Press, 1983.

Putnam, S. M., Stiles, W. B., Jacob, M. C., and James, S. A. "Teaching the Medical Interview: An Intervention Study." *Journal of General Internal Medicine*, 1988, *3*, 38–47.

Quill, T. E. "Recognizing and Adjusting to Barriers in Doctor-Patient Communication." *Annals of Internal Medicine*, 1989, *111*, 51–57.

Quill, T. E., and Townsend, P. "Bad News: Delivery, Dialogue, and Dilemmas." *Archives of Internal Medicine*, 1991, *151*(3), 463–468.

Richards, J., and McDonald, P. "Doctor-Patient Communication in Surgery." *Journal of the Royal Society of Medicine*, 1985, *78*, 922–924.

Root, M. J. "Communication Barriers Between Older Women and Physicians." *Public Health Reports*, 1987, *July-August Supplement*, 152–155.

Rosenbaum, E. E. *The Doctor.* New York: Ballantine Books, 1988.

Roter, D. L., Hall, J. A., and Katz, N. R. "Relations Between Physicians' Behaviors and Analogue Patients' Satisfaction, Recall, and Impressions." *Medical Care*, 1987, *25*, 437–451.

Roter, D. L., Hall, J. A., and Katz, N. R. "Patient-Physician Communication: A Descriptive Summary of the Literature." *Patient Education and Counseling*, 1988, *12*, 99.

Rowland-Morin, P. A., and Carroll, J. G. "Verbal Communication Skills and Patient Satisfaction: A Study of Doctor-Patient Interviews." *Evaluation and the Health Professions*, 1990, *13*, 168–185.

Schain, W. S. "Physician-Patient Communication About Breast Cancer: A Challenge for the 1990's." *Surgical Clinics of North America*, 1990, *70*, 917–936.

Scharf, B. F. "Teaching Patients to Speak Up: Past and Future Trends." *Patient Education and Counseling*, 1988, *11*, 95–108.

Schonwetter, R. S., and others. "Educating the Elderly: Cardiopulmonary Resuscitation Decisions Before and After Intervention." *Journal of the American Geriatrics Society*, 1991, *39*, 372–377.

Seale, C. "Communication and Awareness About Death: A Study of a Random Sample of Dying People." *Social Science and Medicine*, 1991, *32*, 943–952.

Suchman, A. L., and Matthews, D. A. "What Makes the Patient-Doctor Relationship Therapeutic? Exploring the Connexional

Dimension of Medical Care." *Annals of Internal Medicine*, 1988, *108*, 125-130.

Thompson, S. C., Nanni, C., and Schwankovsky, L. "Patient-Oriented Interventions to Improve Communication in a Medical Office Visit." *Health Psychology*, 1990, *9*, 390-404.

Ventres, W., and Gordon, P. "Communication Strategies in Caring for the Underserved." *Journal of Health Care for the Poor and Underserved*, 1990, *1*, 305-314.

Viswanathan, R., Clark, J. J., and Viswanathan, K. "Physicians' and the Public's Attitudes on Communication About Death." *Archives of Internal Medicine*, 1986, *146*, 2029-2033.

Waitzkin, H. "Doctor-Patient Communication: Clinical Implications of Social Scientific Research." *Journal of the American Medical Association*, 1984, *252*, 2441-2446.

Waitzkin, H., and Stoeckle, J. D. "Information Control and the Micropolitics of Health Care: Summary of an Ongoing Research Project." *Social Science and Medicine*, 1976, *10*, 263-276.

Wasserman, R. C., and Inui, T. S. "Systematic Analysis of Clinician-Patient Interactions: A Critique of Recent Approaches with Suggestions for Future Research." *Medical Care*, 1983, *21*, 279-293.

Weisman, C. S. "Communication Between Women and Their Health Care Providers: Research Questions and Unanswered Questions." *Public Health Reports*, 1987, *Jul-Aug Supplement*, 147-151.

Wisiak, U. V., Kroll, W., and List, W. "Communication During the Pre-Operative Visit." *European Journal of Anaesthesiology*, 1991, *6*, 65-68.

Woolley, F. R., Kane, R. L., Hughes, C. C., and Wright, D. D. "The Effects of Doctor-Patient Communication on Satisfaction and Outcome of Care." *Social Science and Medicine*, 1978, *12*, 123-128.

5

Innovations in Patient-Centered Education

Beth Ellers

Patients need information, skills, and support in order to handle the experience of illness and adjust to the rigors of medical treatment. They need to know what to expect. They want to know how their illness will affect their daily lives and how to improve the quality of their lives. If they are to maintain or improve their health in the future, they may need to learn new behaviors and unlearn old ones. "When I left [the hospital]," one patient told us, "I left understanding what took place, what I could expect, what the prognosis was, how I could help myself, which was really the big thing—what I have to do now."

The type of information and support patients want and need will vary, because of both individual and situational differences. Patients with an acute, self-limited illness may need a short-term intervention, with support and information about the disease process, treatment, or procedures. Patients with a chronic condition, on the other hand, may require long-term educational interactions that focus on living with the illness and learning new health-related behaviors. The needs of patients with a chronic illness may also change over time, as they learn more about the illness and its effect on their lives and as their clinical condition changes. Patient education is thus an *interactive* process, distinct from the one-way didactic transfer of information usually associated with patient teaching (Giloth, 1990). Patient education aims to promote an understanding of illness, treatment, and health, and the patient's active participation must be part of this learning process.

Patients who participate in successful educational programs are more satisfied with their health care and express markedly less anxiety (Bartlett, 1989; Devine and Cook, 1986). As one focus-group patient commented, "The unknown is sometimes scarier than what they tell you." Although research has yet to show definitively which programs and approaches work best for which patients, many studies have documented positive outcomes. These outcomes include (1) enhanced knowledge (Beckie, 1989; Brown, 1988), (2) improved adherence to medical regimens (Bailey and others, 1987), (3) improved physical outcomes (Mazzuca, 1982), (4) decreased rates of rehospitalization (Matthes, 1979), and (5) more efficient utilization of health services (Beckie, 1989). Although the overall cost-effectiveness of patient education has yet to be assessed rigorously (Kaplan and Davis, 1986; Webber, 1990), the evidence suggests that successful programs can also reduce institutional costs by shortening lengths of stay, decreasing the rate of complications, and reducing malpractice claims (Bartlett, 1989; "Preop Education . . . ," 1985).

If the benefits of patient involvement and understanding are well documented and widely accepted, why, then, is more not accomplished? The barriers are numerous and are often entrenched in the organizational bureaucracy and the health care system. Within the organization, patient education may rank as a low priority with administration and staff. Lack of coordination among departments and "turf" issues—for example between nurses and physicians—can lead to fragmented approaches to patient education (Webber, 1990). Shortened lengths of stay also leave staff too little time to attend to patients' educational needs, especially when overwhelmed with the medical needs of very sick patients. Also, hospital patients may often be too sick to learn effectively (Armstrong, 1989; Giloth, 1990). Patients in need of ongoing education are often treated as outpatients, where they have limited access to formal educational programs.

Clinicians, primarily physicians and nurses, may also lack the training to be effective educators. The medical model of illness emphasizes pathophysiology, whereas to patients, illness presents a larger *problem of living*. As one of our focus-group participants observed, "Interns and residents are not taught patient care skills; they are taught clinical skills. They're not taught to have interpersonal relationships with the patients. In fact, they're encouraged in subtle ways not to have interpersonal relationships with their patients." Even when patient education is encouraged, providers may not be rewarded for the time they spend in educational efforts. Role models who can effectively integrate an educational approach to patient care into a demanding, crisis-oriented work setting are too often nonexistent (Giloth, 1990; Webber, 1990). Nor do patients always understand the educational role of health care providers. Many view their physician as the only appropriate source of information and do not expect or look for such help from nursing or support staff (Close, 1988). Patients may also be reluctant participants in an interactive process. They may hesitate to ask questions, adopting the passive attitude, "If the doctors thought it was important for me to know, they would have told me."

And finally, the field of patient education is currently limited by the lack of any rigorous understanding of the effectiveness of various educational approaches. We know relatively little about which programs work best for which patients. No single educational method can be applied with cookbook ease to produce an informed, much less a transformed, patient. Changing behavior requires complex strategies, often over time, which may not be equally effective for every patient.

In this chapter, we first examine the components of a patient-centered approach to education, always keeping in mind that it is the patient's perspective that matters. We then turn our attention to intervention strategies and programs that may improve the quality of patient-centered education in an institutional setting.

Components of Patient Education

What do patients need and care most about?

Patients need information, and they need to understand how to incorporate that information into their lives. Patients tell us, first of all, that information is very important to them. As one focus-group patient put it, "What I wanted to see in the hospital was that everything was explained to me—that's number one." Increasing patients' knowledge base is an essential component of most educational programs, and it appears to have a positive effect on adherence to medical regimens (Raleigh and Odtohan, 1987). However, knowledge alone usually does not change behavior or improve adherence. Studies suggest, for example, that while basic nutrition knowledge has increased among the general public, most people do not understand how to apply this knowledge when they select foods and ingredients in the consumer marketplace (Glanz and Mullis, 1988). As important to patients as their clinical understanding of disease processes, then, is knowing how to incorporate health information into their lives. In the words of one focus-group patient, "I would like to be involved as much as possible in my continuing care and to understand it." The degree to which patients want or can participate actively in decision making and learning will vary. To be effective, patient education programs must do *more* than transfer information; they must seek to create an interactive rather than a didactic approach.

How is this accomplished? No single model or type of patient education program has been shown to be superior in effectiveness. Most programs can document some improved outcome. However, programs that address the emotional factors that hinder or promote healthy behaviors and effective coping tend to achieve better results. Successful patient education programs enhance learning through methods such as reinforcement, individualization, and feedback. In a meta-analysis of seventy interventions designed to improve knowledge, adherence to medication regimens, and clinical outcomes in patients with chronic conditions, Mullen, Green, and Persinger (1985) found that individualization, feedback, and reinforcement were the strongest predictors of educational effectiveness. Moreover, programs using a combination of approaches have been shown to be more effective than those relying on a single technique (Haynes, Wang, and Da Mota Gomes, 1987). Involving the family in the educational process has also been shown to be effective.

Patients need to know what to expect. Those dreaded words, "This won't hurt a bit," still evoke fear and anger in many of us. Patients are often not told realistically how much pain or discomfort to expect during hospitalization. Of the patients we surveyed in the Picker/Commonwealth national survey, 21 percent reported that neither the physician nor the nurse explained how much discomfort to expect during a test. Among surgical patients, 23 percent said the surgeon did not tell them how much discomfort they would have, and 22 percent reported that the surgeon did not tell them accurately how they would feel after surgery. Focus-group patients also emphasized the importance of knowing what to expect. They want to know how painful a procedure is likely to be, how long they will stay in the hospital, and if and when they will be able to return to work and to their "normal" life-style.

Patients need different amounts and different kinds of information. While patients recognize their need for information, what they want to know and how much detail they desire vary enormously. Some people handle the stress of illness by mastering every clinical detail; others become intimidated by too much detail. As one focus-group patient expressed it, "I think different people need different amounts of information. *You* need it all. I'm not sure *I* need it all. I need about as much as I'm interested in knowing." How much they are interested in knowing may also change over the course of an illness. The answer may not be clear-cut, even to the patient, as another observed: "I struggled in the hospital, because part of me wanted to know every detail and part of me wanted to forget and just have them take my appendix out, or baby me." Clearly, then, no single informational package is appropriate for every patient. Information that is not tailored to patients' particular needs at a particular time may raise their level of anxiety and thereby do more harm than good.

Patient-centered education addresses the needs, goals, and motivation of the patient, rather than those of the program or provider. If educational plans are to meet the individual needs of the patient, it is the *patient* who must first educate the health care provider. The effectiveness of any individual plan must continually be assessed, not only in terms of what patients learn but also in terms of what they want to learn and how it impacts on their health and their lives. Because the patients' needs and goals are likely to change throughout the course of an illness, this educational assessment must be ongoing.

Patient educators must also bear in mind that the patients' goals may be different from the program's stated goals. Patients referred to a smoking cessation program, for example, may not really wish to stop smoking. In a study of British patients recovering from heart attacks, Murray (1989) found that although most subjects could identify common risk factors for heart disease, such as smoking and obesity, they rarely associated these factors with their own heart attacks. Rather, they blamed overwork, stress, or worry as the cause, even when they were smokers or bearers of a known risk factor. An education program designed to lower the risk of heart disease would therefore have to address the *patient's perceptions* of risk and identify changeable behaviors in order to be effective.

Tailoring educational programs to the patient will also require taking into account cultural differences in health beliefs, language, and communication styles. Non-English-speaking patients may need interpreters or culturally sensitive written or audiovisual material in their native language. Moreover, many patients have difficulty reading, although they may be hesitant to admit the fact and are adept at hiding it.

Patient educational programs must be evaluated from the patient's perspective. In planning a hospital-based program, educators must clarify program goals in terms of patients' needs, identify appropriate measurable outcomes, and build in the capacity for ongoing evaluation and adaptation. Different types of educational programs will have different goals. A preoperative educational program, for example, may strive to increase the patient's knowledge, inform the patient about what to expect before, during, and after surgery, and relieve anxiety. A cardiac rehabilitation program might aim to reduce cardiac risk factors through life-style modification programs targeting smoking, diet, exercise, stress reduction, or long-term psychological adjustment. Some programs—for instance, those designed to decrease lengths of stay or reduce the number of unreimbursable readmissions—may be designed primarily to serve the hospital's interests, rather than those of the patient. Yet the ultimate success of any program will be determined by its ability to meet patients' needs. Patients are therefore the best source of evidence about a program's outcomes and should be included in the planning and evaluation process.

Patients also need information and education when they are not in the hospital. For patients with an acute, self-limiting illness, a short-term in-hospital educational program may be appropriate. But most patients these days are hospitalized for acute episodes of a chronic illness that requires continuous treatment. Patient education programs, too, need to bridge the gap between hospital and community, to promote the long-term care of the chronically ill.

While they are in the hospital, patients are sick and anxious. They are preoccupied by worries about survival, pain, and discomfort, and their goal is to be discharged. Circumstances such as these are not conducive to learning. Patients discharged "quicker and sicker" have less time for in-hospital education, and they are less receptive to learning. Yet optimal treatment of chronic illness may require long-term adherence to medical regimens as well as long-term behavior change. More complex care requires more complex educational efforts and continuing interaction between health care provider, the patient, and the patient's family. These efforts must also be sensitive to the patient's changing needs. It is unrealistic to expect a single educational session to accomplish long-lasting behavior change with an improved health outcome (Oberst, 1989; Windsor, Green, and Roseman, 1980).

Although providing support services for patients after discharge may not be within a hospital's traditional scope of responsibility, the hospital is the health care institution to which patients traditionally turn for support, and it may be the *only* health care institution in the community with the resources to meet the long-term educational needs of chronic patients. A hospital's need to reduce the number of uncompensated days of inpatient care may also add the incentive to do so.

Patient education requires planning and commitment throughout the organization. Some health care providers think of patient education as handing a pamphlet to a patient or turning on a closed-circuit television. Even those who recognize their broader educational role may have to forfeit it in the face of competing crises. If educational efforts are to be pursued more thoroughly and more rigorously, they must be given higher priority throughout the organization, and this message must come from the top.

Successful patient educational programs require organizational support in the form of financial and staffing resources and innovative policies. This, in turn, entails a comprehensive planning process and not merely hiring a patient educator. The effort must be both systematic and operational throughout the organization. Such a commitment will ensure that patient education is not placed on the back burner because of competing work pressures. Staff must be rewarded for their patient educational efforts. Hospital administrators can promote patient education in a variety of ways. The administration can provide overall direction and establish a centralized, interdisciplinary committee to set policy and oversee patient educational efforts. Patient education can be incorporated into the hospital's strategic objectives, and a hospital policy statement can be issued to strengthen the organization's commitment. The administration can also ensure adequate budget support for implementation (Bartlett, 1989). Strategies to enhance patient education may include developing and refining existing programs; developing new programs, where there is already a high level of demonstrated interest; performing communitywide or institutional needs assessment (Breckon, 1982); and promoting training programs for health care professionals to strengthen their role as educators.

Financial constraints are a frequent inhibitor of innovation (Kaplan and Davis, 1986). However, third-party payers may cover some patient education costs when they are ordered by a physician. Some patients are also willing to pay extra out-of-pocket expenses for educational services they view as a high priority (Sumpmann and Goldstein, 1991). Moreover, promoting patient education does not require a radical restructuring of the organization or a tremendous financial commitment. The University of Minnesota Hospital has developed an innovative hands-on program to teach patients and family members caregiving skills. The program uses only one patient education specialist, who serves as a resource and consultant to clinical staff; they in turn develop the educational materials.

Innovations in Patient Education: Strategies and Programs

Many innovative approaches to patient education incorporating the basic principles outlined in this chapter have been developed at hospitals throughout the country. We describe some of them here, not to endorse any particular program but to suggest the interesting range of ideas and conceptual approaches.

Expanding Access to Informational Resources

Many programs have sought to enhance patient education by making a broad variety of educational resources more accessible to patients and their families. At the Planetree Resource Center in San Francisco, for example, information on virtually every medical condition or diagnostic and therapeutic procedure is either on hand or accessible to anyone who inquires. This includes both literature written for laypeople and medical scientific publications that are usually available only in medical libraries. The center also gathers information on nonmedical or social support services and on alternative and experimental methods of treatment and healing. It is open to the public, supported by fees from its research services, memberships, and contributions. It serves a national clientele, responding to written and telephone, as well as walk-in, inquiries.

The M. D. Anderson Cancer Center at the University of Texas in Houston also maintains a patient and family resource center in an adjacent hotel, where outpatients and families stay during treatment. This resource center supports and augments M. D. Anderson's extensive patient education classes. Within each clinical area of the center, a multidisciplinary patient education committee area is responsible for assessing the needs of patients and family members, designing interventions for all stages of illness, and monitoring quality (Villejo, Giloth, and Zerbe, 1988).

The Ohio State University Hospitals have developed structured interdisciplinary patient education programs in thirty separate clinical areas, including preoperative education, diabetes, bone marrow transplant, and cardiac rehabilitation, according to the hospital's patient education department. Here, too, multidisciplinary teams develop the educational programs, spelling out the goals and objectives of each, team member responsibilities, and operating mechanics. The patient education department teaches the staff to teach patients. Education has become part of the job description for the hospital's clinical staff.

Health education staff at Northern California Kaiser Permanente are studying ways to enhance patient education through pamphlet rack placement, the development and dissemination of a core pamphlet collection for primary care, the use of commissioned art to stimulate questions and educational interchange with providers, and the use of consumer-accessed video programs in waiting areas (Giloth, 1990).

The Beth Israel Hospital in Boston has tried to find ways to use patients themselves as an educational resource. The hospital's peer support program, "Patient-to-Patient, Heart-to-Heart," pairs patients who have received cancer treatment with newly diagnosed patients one-on-one to share information and emotional support. Volunteers are carefully screened and trained. After the initial contact, patients set the agenda and the frequency of contact based on their own needs, according to the program coordinator.

Interactive videodiscs are a vehicle to inform patients about treatment options for a variety of conditions, such as low-back pain and prostate cancer. The interactive format allows patients to get information tailored to their symptoms and to skip or repeat. A videodisc on early breast cancer produced by the Foundation for Informed Medical Decision Making exemplifies the *shared-decision model*. Treatment options are discussed, with emphasis on the importance of the patient's choice and feelings. Women who have undergone treatment discuss the reasons for their choices on screen (Faltermayer, 1992).

Enhancing Patient Participation

Patient educational programs have been found to be more effective when behavioral or psychosocial needs are addressed, along with cognitive ones. This more comprehensive approach makes education more relevant to patients' lives and also involves them more in the educational process. At Beth Israel Hospital in Newark, New Jersey, the patient contract is used to enhance patient involvement on an inpatient basis. Each patient's primary nurse initiates a discussion of nursing care needs, negotiates with the patient about the respective responsibilities of the patient, family, and nurse, and draws up a contract that reflects these negotiations. The contract approach is designed to individualize the care delivery process and establish clear lines of communication in an interactive style.

Brookhaven Memorial Hospital Medical Center in Patchogue, New York, developed an education and counseling program to meet the informational, educational, and psychosocial needs of cancer patients and their families. A psychologist and a nurse educator provided both inpatient and outpatient education and counseling services, depending on the individual needs of the patient and family. Education and counseling formats varied, being group or individual, short-term or long-term. A major component of the project entailed educating and training health care professionals on approaches to patient education (Lane and Liss-Levinson, 1980). Although the program has been discontinued, this concept merits recognition for its patient-centered approach.

The Cancer Education and Prevention Center at Summit Medical Center (formerly Samuel Merritt Hospital) in Oakland, California, is a cancer screening clinic that teaches patients self-examination and surveillance techniques, assesses risk factors for cancer, and develops plans for life-style and behavior changes to reduce risk. The center offers both community classes and individual education and screening. To establish a better rapport with community physicians, it provides professional education classes and lectures and otherwise tries to address physicians' needs as well as those of patients (Schweitzer, 1988). The center relies heavily on volunteers and community support to keep costs down, according to staff.

The Wholistic Health Center project in Hinsdale, Illinois, started as a church-based family practice medical care facility. An interdisciplinary team of physicians, pastoral counselors, and nurses addressed all aspects of an individual's health needs, including the spiritual and emotional, disease prevention and health promotion, and methods of confronting and coping with life's stresses. On entering the program, each patient participated in a twenty-minute health planning conference with the interdisciplinary team, designed to assess health needs, identify sources of stress, and promote patient participation in the holistic approach. Patients were encouraged to repeat this health conference at least yearly. The Wholistic Health Center also offered health screening and promotion programs and support groups (Tubesing, Holinger, Westberg, and Lichter, 1977). In recent years, however, difficulty recruiting new staff physicians has forced the center to shift its focus from the holistic practice of medicine to psychosocial counseling.

Integrating Health Care into the Patient's Life-Style

Translating knowledge and cognitive understanding into practice, for patients who want and need to change harmful behaviors, can be difficult. The Maricopa County General Hospital in Phoenix, Arizona, developed a diabetic day care center to help patients adjust to the diagnosis of diabetes and the life-style modification it requires. The center was designed to provide an environment for diabetes education outside of the artificial setting of the hospital. Insulin-dependent diabetic patients visit the outpatient day-care center for five days of education and treatment and follow up afterward according to their individual needs and progress. The center's educational efforts reportedly resulted in significantly reduced days of hospitalization (Matthes, 1979). Medicaid and Medicare will reimburse for the educational services, while other third-party payers will partially cover costs.

Designed for rehabilitation education, "Easy Street" at Phoenix Memorial Hospital in Phoenix, Arizona, is a mock village or shopping area that allows disabled patients to practice living skills in a realistic but protected environment. The bank, grocery store, bar and grill, movie theater, bus stop, laundromat, and outdoor cafe all present typical situations and obstacles that patients encounter on the outside. Aimed initially at assisting elderly patients with perambulatory problems, this program has since expanded to include rehabilitation patients with a variety of disabilities ("Rehab Program . . . ," 1985). Patients and staff have enjoyed this practical approach to rehabilitation.

As an adjunct to nutrition education in a hospital setting, Rochester Methodist Hospital in Rochester, Minnesota, provides a Nutrition Education and Dining (NED) cafeteria with low-fat foods and a dietician to help patients and family members select foods most appropriate to individual diet plans (Giloth, 1990). An exam-

ple of a community-based approach to diet modification, the
"Heart-Smart Choices" program at Skagit Valley Hospital and
Health Center in Mount Vernon, Washington, encourages local
restaurants to offer substitutions for high-fat menu items. A hospital dietician evaluates the restaurant's menu and offers recommendations and training to promote healthy alternatives (American
Hospital Association, 1990). Minnesota Heart Health, a similar
community-based program, tries to promote healthy nutrition behavior through its "Dining à la Heart" program. Program staff
work with local restaurants to identify healthy foods on the menu
and with supermarkets to identify and label low-fat and low-sodium
products on the shelves (Glanz and Mullis, 1988).

The University of Alabama at Birmingham's asthma self-
management education program uses a self-care workbook to help
patients learn to live with asthma. The workbook, *Learn Asthma
Control in 7 Days,* was developed to improve patients' cognitive
skills, encourage their daily self-assessment, reinforce their successes, and promote more effective social support. The intervention
also includes a one-to-one counseling session with a health educator, an ongoing asthma support group, and follow-up telephone
calls from the health educator for reinforcement (Bailey and others,
1987). The arthritis self-management course offered by the Stanford
Medical Center in California is a community-based patient educational course that follows detailed protocols to help patients live
with this chronic disease. The course is taught by trained lay leaders, most of whom live with arthritis themselves. Topics covered
include managing symptoms, designing exercise programs, communicating with family and with physicians, and managing anger,
fatigue, and depression. Course participants reportedly have experienced reduced pain, increased levels of physical activity, and less
need for outpatient visits.

Integrating Education into the Health Care System

While many organizations want to promote patient education, competing work pressures and demands may inhibit them. Several interesting approaches have been developed to enhance and protect the
educational component of care. At the Cooperative Care Unit at New

York University Medical Center in New York City, patient education is central to a system of hospital care that relies on patient participation and family involvement. On admission, the patient and a designated care partner are assessed in the education center even before the patient is examined and worked up physically. A multidisciplinary team of nurse educators, nutritionists, social workers, and pharmacists addresses the patient's educational needs through individual instruction and group sessions. Audiovisual and printed material supplement the classes (Grieco, 1991).

While Cooperative Care entails a radical restructuring of hospital care, the Mayo Clinic of Rochester, Minnesota, has developed a simpler way to integrate education into the existing ordering and scheduling system. The clinic has designed disease-specific patient educational courses, which it lists on the standardized physician order form along with all other diagnostic and therapeutic procedures. Every such test or course ordered is automatically scheduled through the clinic's centralized scheduling process within an hour or two of the initial consultation. This approach serves not only to give equal symbolic weight to the educational component of treatment, but it streamlines what might otherwise be a cumbersome referral process.

Patient and Family Skills Training

The Learning Center at the University of Minnesota Hospital and Clinic in Minneapolis offers patients and their families a teaching laboratory where they can learn and practice highly technical skills and procedures. The center is a hands-on laboratory environment, complete with life-sized mannequins and equipment for skills demonstration and practice. This resource is available to patients and families on referral and helps to prepare them for discharge home (Sumpmann, 1989).

Training Staff

Patient-centered care sometimes requires a staff-centered approach, since many health professionals lack basic training in educational methods. Devine and others (1988) showed when surgical staff nurses were given training workshops teaching educational and psychosocial support skills, their patients admitted for elective surgical procedures had shorter lengths of stay and required less medication. The program involved a three-hour two-stage training workshop, plus one hour of additional nurse staff time per hospital stay, and was evaluated to be cost-effective.

The staff education department of Rochester Methodist Hospital in Rochester, Minnesota, also emphasizes the importance of teaching teachers to teach. Nursing orientation and required staff courses of instruction focus on the adult learner and on how people learn when they are sick. In Charlottesville, Virginia, the University of Virginia's Help Communications Project for Low Literacy Patient Education includes a training course called "Say It Simply" to help staff develop materials for low-literacy patients. According to the patient education department, the patient's bill of rights and other educational materials ranging from nutrition to medication information have been revised for low-literacy understanding.

The People Activated Toward Health (PATH) program at South Nassau Communities Hospital in Oceanside, New York, uses older volunteers as an educational resource for health promotion and disease prevention. After completing a training course, volunteers provide supervised screening services and teach their peers about health promotion and the appropriate use of medical services. The program works on two levels: helping volunteers take better care of their own health, while they also educate their peers (American Hospital Association, 1990).

Promoting Cultural Sensitivity

Patients with different cultural backgrounds have different educational needs. The Episcopal Hospital of Philadelphia offers innovative support to its Hispanic population through its patient-liaison programs. The patient-liaison program provides an interpreter for Spanish-speaking patients and their families and a Spanish-English communications guide focusing on key medical and health-related words and phrases. In addition, the program offers Spanish classes to hospital employees. The hospital's community outreach initiatives also include participation in such civic activities as community cleanup programs and career days, high school equivalency diploma classes, and voter registration drives (American Hospital Association, 1990).

Specific programs may also be developed to target the specific needs of different populations. In an effort to meet the needs of the estimated 60,000 to 150,000 undocumented Salvadorans and Guatemalans residing in San Francisco, for example, the Refugee and Immigrant Health Task Force was established to advise the city's Health Commission. San Francisco General Hospital, the city's public hospital, contributed both staff and material support to this interagency effort. Activities included a conference for health care providers, social service workers, and law enforcement personnel, as well as Spanish and English guidebooks listing health care services available for undocumented Latinos. The interagency effort also included mandated sensitivity training for eligibility and registration personnel at San Francisco General Hospital, to acquaint them with the particular problems of undocumented refugees, and an examination of the impact of hospital billing and eligibility procedures on refugee patients. In addition, an outreach campaign was conducted to inform the Latino community of the services and public financial assistance available to undocumented residents and amnesty applicants. This coordinated effort won San Francisco General Hospital top honors in the 1989 California Association of Public Hospitals' Innovator's Award.

The American Indian Health Care Association has developed a *Promoting Healthy Traditions Workbook: A Guide to the Healthy People 2000 Campaign* (Scott, 1990), which provides programmatic models and resource information for community-based health care for Native Americans. The association has also published the *Native American Health Promotion and Disease Prevention Bibliography* (1990), which outlines health promotion projects in Native American communities. The Native American Research and Training Center in Tucson, Arizona, has produced culturally sensitive educational videotapes and monographs on diabetes and holistic health care targeting Native Americans and Alaskans. Topics include government policies, specific health and rehabilitation problems affecting Native Americans, and cultural issues relating to Indian concepts of health, disease, and disability.

Facilitating Continuity of Care

Many health educational programs promote continuity of care by helping to bridge the gap between hospital and community. Canadian patients recovering from coronary artery bypass graft surgery have access to a supportive-educative telephone program, which puts them in regular contact with a cardiac rehabilitation nurse specialist during the six to eight weeks following hospitalization. This telephone follow-up has been especially important for people living in remote areas of Alberta. Home visits are made in some situations. The educational content of the program includes information on coronary artery disease, self-care measures, and treatment regimens. This low-cost program saves money through picking up potential complications early (Beckie, 1989). The GENESIS Health Center for Women and Children at Tampa General Hospital in Florida won a 1990 Safety Net Award from the National Association of Public Hospitals for its coordinated, patient-oriented approach to outpatient and inpatient care. This comprehensive program offers a wide variety of services, such as outreach and case management, gynecological and obstetrical care, child health care, nutritional counseling, health education, social services, and financial assistance (Gage, 1991). Additional examples of transitional and continuing care programs are discussed in Chapter Nine.

Teaching Aids

Because patients have individual styles of learning, a combination of teaching methods is often more effective than any single technique alone (Haynes, Wang, and Da Mota Gomes, 1987; Windsor, Green, and Roseman, 1980). A brief description of a variety of teaching aids follows.

Audiovisual methods, especially videotapes, are increasing in popularity. They can be relatively inexpensive to produce, provide more consistent information, and have the potential to reach a larger audience than one-on-one teaching. They are also especially useful for nonliterate patient populations, child and adult. Videotapes for home use can replicate and reinforce information given to the patient during earlier clinical encounters. Dramatic role modeling is particularly effective in this medium and has been shown to increase patients' knowledge, improve their coping skills, and decrease anxiety in stressful situations (Gagliano, 1988).

Contracts have been used successfully with outpatients who have complex care needs or who must attempt to modify entrenched behaviors. The process of negotiation between health care provider and patient produces a written document specifying learning behaviors, teaching methodologies, responsibilities of the teacher and the learner, and methods of follow-up and evaluation (Armstrong, 1989; Haynes, Wang, and Da Mota Gomes, 1987; Windsor, Green, and Roseman, 1980). A variation on this method is the "wellness prescription," modified from the U.S. Army's "Be Alive in 2005" program. This form, designed to encourage self-care, includes risk factors that should be modified, exercise treatment, nutritional guidelines, stress management ideas, and recommended reading (Fletcher, 1985).

Self-monitoring diaries are also designed to encourage patients to practice self-management skills on a continuing basis, increasing their sense of responsibility and participation and reinforcing learning (Bailey and others, 1987). *Role playing and dramatization* enhance patients' understanding and interest through simulated learning situations (Breckon, 1982). *Individualized printed handouts,* with relevant information circled or handwritten in, add emphasis to the message. Take-home materials, such as medication cards, can be individualized to encourage integration of the information (Giloth, 1990). *Bedside bulletin boards* allow patients and families to keep track of questions or progress during hospitalization (Giloth, 1990).

The *self-care movement* offers an alternative approach to patient education, in which the experienced patient, rather than the physician or health care professional, is the primary health resource (Fletcher, 1985). In general, self-help groups share the following characteristics: a shared common experience among members, mutual help and support, a faith in collective willpower and belief, an emphasis on information, and constructive action toward shared goals (Robinson, 1978). Self-care programs have reported success in increasing health knowledge and effective positive behavior changes, as well as in teaching patients self-care practices. The St.

Paul Helping Hand Health Center in St. Paul, Minnesota, recognizes the shared responsibility of provider and patient through its patient library and self-care classes (Fletcher, 1985). (The center recently underwent a reorganization because of a merger with United Family Practice.) According to the New Jersey Self-Help Clearing House, the demand for self-help groups has skyrocketed in recent years. Established to help New Jersey residents locate self-help groups in their own area, the clearinghouse's mission has expanded to help callers establish their own mutual support groups where none is locally available. Clearinghouse staff and volunteers have assisted in the formation of an estimated 550 new groups in the past eight years (Ferguson, 1992).

Summary

Patient-centered education recognizes the importance of patients' and families' informed participation in their continuing health care. To be successful, patient-centered education requires a multilevel organizational commitment. Health education should not be limited to the in-hospital setting. Strategies to enhance patient education include expanding access to educational resources, enhancing patient participation, integrating health care into the patient's life-style, integrating education into the health care system, providing patient and family skills training and training for professional staff, promoting cultural sensitivity, and facilitating continuity of care. Comprehensive approaches employing a variety of methods and strategies are most effective and must include ongoing assessment of the patient's needs and goals.

Suggestions for Improvement

- Assess the patient's educational needs, together with clinical needs, on admission to the hospital.
- Include patient education classes and support services on standard physicians' order forms and schedule them as methodically as diagnostic tests and procedures.
- Offer a teaching laboratory environment with equipment for patients and families to learn and practice technical skills.

- Negotiate contracts with patients that outline the care plan, educational goals and behaviors, teaching methodologies, and respective responsibilities of patient and health care provider.
- Individualize printed educational materials, using circled or filled-in information, to provide specific instructions for each patient.
- Offer culturally sensitive educational materials tailored to specific ethnic groups served by your health care institution.
- Follow patients discharged from the hospital with an educational telephone program, providing information on disease processes, self-care, treatment, and health promotion.
- Provide self-care workbooks or self-monitoring diaries to encourage self-assessment and reinforce learning.
- Set up an outpatient educational center for education, support, and treatment, which allows patients to learn at their own pace.
- Write a "wellness prescription," which includes health-related behaviors that need to be modified, exercise regimens, nutritional guidelines, stress management ideas, and recommended reading.
- Use experienced patients as teachers to share information and offer support.
- Train volunteers in health promotion and disease prevention to assist in patient education courses and health screening programs.
- Provide workshops for professional staff to clarify their educational role, discuss alternative teaching methodologies, and reinforce psychosocial skills.
- Form multidisciplinary patient education committees in various clinical areas to assess the needs of patients and family members, design interventions, and evaluate progress. Include patients and family members on these committees.

References

American Hospital Association. *Healthy People 2000: America's Hospitals Respond.* Chicago: American Hospital Association, 1990.

American Indian Health Care Association. *Native American Health*

Promotion and Disease Prevention Bibliography. St. Paul, Minn.: American Indian Health Care Association, 1990.

Armstrong, M. L. "Orchestrating the Process of Patient Education: Methods and Approaches." *Nursing Clinics of North America,* 1989, *24*(3), 597–604.

Bailey, W. C., and others. "Promoting Self-Management in Adults with Asthma: An Overview of the UAB Program." *Health Education Quarterly,* 1987, *14*(3), 345–355.

Bartlett, E. E. "Patient Education Can Lower Costs, Improve Quality." *Hospitals,* 1989, *63*(21), 88.

Beckie, T. "A Supportive-Educative Telephone Program: Impact on Knowledge and Anxiety after CABG Surgery." *Heart & Lung,* 1989, *18*(1), 46–55.

Breckon, D. J. *Hospital Health Education.* Rockville, Md.: Aspen Systems Corporation, 1982.

Brown, S. A. "Effects of Educational Interventions in Diabetes Care: A Meta-Analysis of Findings." *Nursing Research,* 1988, *37*(4), 223–230.

Close, A. "Patient Education: A Literature Review." *Journal of Advanced Nursing,* 1988, *13*, 203–213.

Devine, E. C., and Cook, T. D. "Clinical and Cost-Saving Effects of Psychoeducational Interventions with Surgical Patients: A Meta-Analysis." *Research in Nursing and Health,* 1986, *9*, 89–105.

Devine, E. C., and others. "Clinical and Financial Effects of Psychoeducational Care Provided to Adult Surgical Patients in the Post-DRG Environment." *American Journal of Public Health,* 1988, *78*(10), 1293–1297.

Faltermayer, E. "Let's Really Cure the Health Care System." *Fortune,* Mar. 23, 1992, pp. 46–58.

Ferguson, T. "Patient, Heal Thyself." *The Futurist,* 1992, 9–13.

Fletcher, D. J. "Self-Care: How to Help Patients Share Responsibility for Their Health." *Postgraduate Medicine,* 1985, *78*(2), 213–223.

Gage, L. S. *America's Safety Net Hospitals: The Foundation of Our Nation's Health System.* Washington, D.C.: National Association of Public Hospitals, 1991.

Gagliano, M. E. "A Literature Review on the Efficacy of Video in

Patient Education." *Journal of Medical Education,* 1988, *63,* 785-792.

Giloth, B. E. "Promoting Patient Involvement: Educational, Organizational, and Environmental Strategies." *Patient Education and Counseling,* 1990, *15,* 29-38.

Glanz, K., and Mullis, R. M. "Environmental Interventions to Promote Healthy Eating: A Review of Models, Programs, and Evidence." *Health Education Quarterly,* 1988, *15*(4), 395-415.

Grieco, A. J. "Cooperative Care Smooths Transition Home." *Picker/Commonwealth Report,* 1991, *1*(1), 8.

Haynes, R. B., Wang, E., and Da Mota Gomes, M. "A Critical Review of Interventions to Improve Compliance with Prescribed Medications." *Patient Education and Counseling,* 1987, *10,* 155-166.

Kaplan, R. M., and Davis, W. K. "Evaluating the Costs and Benefits of Outpatient Diabetes Education and Nutrition Counseling." *Diabetes Care,* 1986, *9*(1), 81-86.

Lane, D. S., and Liss-Levinson, W. "Education and Counselling for Cancer Patients: Lifting the Shroud of Silence." *Patient Counseling and Health Education,* 1980, *2*(4), 154-160.

Matthes, M. L. "Beyond the Hospital: Diabetic Day Care." *American Journal of Nursing,* 1979, *79*(1), 105-106.

Mazzuca, S. A. "Does Patient Education in Chronic Disease Have Therapeutic Value?" *Journal of Chronic Diseases,* 1982, *35,* 521-529.

Mullen, P. D., Green, L. W., and Persinger, G. S. "Clinical Trials of Patient Education for Chronic Conditions: A Comparative Meta-Analysis of Intervention Types." *Preventive Medicine,* 1985, *14,* 753-781.

Murray, P. J. "Rehabilitation Information and Health Beliefs in the Post-Coronary Patient: Do We Meet Their Information Needs?" *Journal of Advanced Nursing,* 1989, *14,* 686-693.

Oberst, M. T. "Perspectives on Research in Patient Teaching." *Nursing Clinics of North America,* 1989, *24*(3), 621-628.

"Preop Education Can Cut LOS and Cost, Aid PPS Delivery." *Hospitals,* 1985, *59*(4), 78, 80, 82.

Raleigh, E. H., and Odtohan, B. C. "The Effect of a Cardiac Teaching Program on Patient Rehabilitation." *Heart & Lung,* 1987, *13*(3), 311–317.

"Rehab Program Brings Patients to Life on 'Easy Street.'" *Hospitals,* 1985, *59*(16), 122.

Robinson, D. "Self-Help Groups." *British Journal of Hospital Medicine,* 1978, *20*(3), 306–311.

Schweitzer, R. J. "A Cancer Education and Prevention Center: A Community Program." *Cancer,* 1988, *62,* 1821–1822.

Scott, S. *Promoting Healthy Traditions Workbook: A Guide to the Healthy People 2000 Campaign.* St. Paul, Minn.: American Indian Health Care Association, 1990.

Sumpmann, M. "An Education Center For Patients' High-Tech Learning Needs." *Patient Education and Counseling,* 1989, *13,* 309–323.

Sumpmann, M., and Goldstein, N. "Patient Learning Center: A Model for Discharge Skills Training." *Picker/Commonwealth Report,* 1991, *1*(1), 10–11.

Tubesing, D. A., Holinger, P. C., Westberg, G. E., and Lichter, E. A. "The Wholistic Health Center Project: An Action Research Health Care at the Primary Level." *Medical Care,* 1977, *15*(3), 217–227.

Villejo, L. A., Giloth, B. E., and Zerbe, D. A. "Patient Education Services." In S. Nathanson and D. Lerman (eds.), *Outpatient Cancer Centers: Implementation and Management.* Chicago: American Hospital Publishing, 1988.

Webber, G. C. "Patient Education: A Review of the Issues." *Medical Care,* 1990, *28*(11), 1089–1103.

Windsor, R. A., Green, L. W., and Roseman, J. M. "Health Promotion and Maintenance for Patients with Chronic Obstructive Pulmonary Disease: A Review." *Journal of Chronic Diseases,* 1980, *33,* 5–12.

6

Enhancing
Physical Comfort

Janice D. Walker

Sick people need to be taken care of. Long before hospitals became gleaming citadels of space-age medicine, this caring function was their primary reason for being. And whatever the criteria doctors, insurance companies, or government officials may now use to justify a hospital admission, patients still look to hospitals to give them the basic physical care they cannot give themselves. "It seems like they can do almost everything outside the hospital now," one focus-group patient remarked. "I guess the reason you really have to be there is so they can watch you and take care of you." Patients will forgive hospitals and health professionals many things, but they will not forgive their dereliction in performing this fundamental task.

The hospital stays of most patients can be divided into two phases: an acute phase, involving either an invasive procedure or the exacerbation of a medical condition, and a healing and repair phase. Besides giving patients needed medical treatment, the job of the hospital is to minimize the physical trauma of the first phase and (notwithstanding today's shortened lengths of stay) to maximize comfort and healing in the second. In this chapter, we address, in turn, three principal aspects of this task, based on what patients

Note: The author gratefully acknowledges the helpful comments of Annette M. Delaney and Peggy Reilly in the preparation of this chapter.

tell us to be most important to their physical comfort: controlling acute pain—in many respects, the most immediate requirement of medical care; providing what we might call basic nursing care to support and maintain normal body functions; and minimizing the stresses of the hospital's physical environment to provide a supportive atmosphere for healing and recovery.

Acute Pain Management

Before the introduction of anesthesia, pain was an inevitable by-product of surgery, childbirth, and many illnesses. Nineteenth-century medical literature is rich with almost unendurably vivid descriptions of pain, as suggested by the following description of a patient undergoing repair of a dislocated hip: "Big drops of perspiration, started by the excess of agony, bestrew the patient's forehead, sharp screams burst from him in peal after peal—all his struggles to free himself and escape the horrid torture are valueless, for he is in the powerful hands of men then as inexorable as death. . . . At last the agony becomes too great for human endurance, and with a wild, despairing yell, the sufferer relapses into unconsciousness" (quoted in Pernick, 1983, p. 26). But nowadays, pain is not inevitable. With the development of anesthesia and advances in the use of narcotics and other analgesics, pain is a manageable aspect of illness and treatment. While it is not desirable to eliminate all pain (since it can often aid in diagnosis or in monitoring a patient's course), the most basic element of the caring function of medicine is the relief of pain, and aggressive pain management is essential to patient-centered care.

And yet, sadly, pain continues to be one of the most feared and debilitating aspects of illness and medical treatment. In the early 1970s, Marks and Sachar (1973) were inspired to study the treatment of pain in medical inpatients as a result of their experience with their hospital's psychosomatic liaison service. They found that psychiatrists were often called to see medical patients described as having severe "emotional" responses to pain, in spite of having been treated with narcotics. What the psychiatrists often found, however, were *not* psychologically disturbed patients or malingerers exaggerating their need for narcotics, but patients in severe

pain because of serious, often life-threatening illness who were receiving far less narcotics than would be required to relieve their
pain. Later, when they conducted structured patient interviews for
the study, Marks and Sachar found that 73 percent of medical patients were in fact enduring moderate to severe distress in spite of
their pain control regimens. Other studies confirmed the undertreatment of pain. Cohen (1980) found that 75 percent of the postoperative patients surveyed experienced moderate or severe pain.
Keeri-Szanto and Heaman (1972) found that 20 percent of surgery
patients were getting inadequate pain relief from conventional intramuscular medications. In 1983, 41 percent of the postoperative
patients questioned by Weis and colleagues said they experienced
moderate to severe pain even with narcotics.

Nor is this situation improving, in spite of the recent development of more effective technology for managing pain. In a disturbing study published in 1987, Donovan, Dillon, and McGuire
found that 58 percent of randomly selected medical and surgical
patients who had pain at some time during their hospitalization
reported having "horrible" or "excruciating" pain at some point,
and only one-third of patients with pain reported obtaining total
relief at any time. Sixty-one percent had been awakened by their
pain. More than two-thirds of the medical and surgical patients
interviewed in our 1989 national patient survey recalled experiencing pain while they were hospitalized, and 86 percent of them described that pain as moderate or severe. Eighteen percent of these
patients also felt that much of their pain could have been eliminated
through "prompt attention of the hospital staff." In 1990, 40 percent of hysterectomy and cholecystectomy patients questioned by
Kuhn found the postoperative experience to be "very painful." Seventy percent of patients in intensive care units interviewed by Puntillo (1990) recalled having pain while they were in the ICU, and
nearly two-thirds described it as moderate or severe.

Perhaps as a result of this experience, patients appear to have
low expectations about pain relief. Only 18 percent of the patients
in one study reported their pain control as inadequate, even though
41 percent of them were in moderate to severe pain (Weis and others,
1983). Donovan (1983) found 31 percent of postoperative patients
felt they got insufficient pain relief, but only 14 percent were dis-

satisfied with their pain control. Puntillo found that most ICU patients neither expected nor received total pain relief. Only 6 percent of patients with pain in the Picker/Commonwealth survey thought they received too little pain medication, even though 86 percent described their pain as moderate or severe. It is sad to think that patients view pain as the rule rather than the exception in medical care. Though they expect state-of-the-art technology in the diagnosis and management of their illness, they accept treatment of pain as it was twenty or more years ago. Patients endure more pain than is necessary. *And yet we have the means to make them comfortable.*

The Challenge of Pain Control

Pain is a highly subjective experience, and many factors complicate its management. Optimal treatment entails multiple steps, beginning with the individual's awareness of pain and effective communication with a clinician about it, the clinician's accurate clinical assessment, and, finally, the administration of appropriate therapy to impart prompt relief.

Individual differences in pain thresholds and responses to pain make objective assessment difficult and complicate pain management (Beecher, 1956; Weis and others, 1983; Lim and others, 1983; Teske, Daut, and Cleeland, 1983; Baer, Davitz, and Lieb, 1970). In a fascinating study published in 1956, Beecher compared the gravity of wounds in military and civilian surgical patients with their reports of pain. Though the wounds inflicted during battle were far more extensive, only one-third of the soldiers requested morphine, and their moods were notable for their "optimistic, even cheerful, state of mind." For the soldiers, their wounds meant sudden release from the terrors of the battlefield. In contrast, 83 percent of the civilian surgical patients wanted morphine, though the surgical trauma was less severe. For these patients, surgery represented a crisis. Beecher concluded that the perceived severity of pain is largely dependent on its meaning to the patient.

Objective assessment of pain is further complicated by the fact that people communicate in different ways about their pain due to cultural influences and individual differences. Some patients verbalize compelling accounts of their pain, while others endure even severe pain in stoic silence. Some assertively demand medication as soon as they notice discomfort, while others wait until pain becomes unbearable before self-consciously requesting relief. Some patients deny wanting medication because they do not want to appear weak or dependent on narcotics, especially in today's "Just-Say-No-to-Drugs" environment (Max, 1990). Some do not want to "bother" the nurse. Patients' difficulties in communicating effectively about pain are further compounded if they speak a different language than the clinician, or if they are unable to speak at all as a result of their illness or treatment (for example, when an endotracheal tube is present).

Just as patients differ in the way they communicate about pain, individual providers differ in their assessment skills. Some investigators have found that providers attribute more pain to patients who can verbalize about it (Baer, Davitz, and Lieb, 1970; Graffam, 1981). But not all patients verbalize, and special skills may be required to assess pain in those who do not. The severity of pain patients experience may be related to factors such as their relationship with their nurses or doctors (Diers, Schmidt, McBride, and Davis, 1972; Egbert, Battit, Welch, and Bartlett, 1964), their sense of control over their pain (Keeri-Szanto, 1979), and their level of anxiety. Evaluating these aspects of pain and intervening effectively to manage them thus may require very sophisticated skills.

Clinicians' attitudes about pain also differ. Total pain relief may not be a nurse's goal in treating a patient, for example (Cohen, 1980). In a study of fifty-two nurses who administered narcotics to control the pain of cancer patients in their care, Rankin and Snider (1984) found that 89 percent believed that their patients were receiving "adequate" medication, even though 67 percent assessed the patients still to be in "moderate" pain. For over half the nurses (58 percent), the stated goal was to reduce pain rather than to relieve it. Another investigator found that only 20 percent of surveyed house staff and nurses sought complete pain relief as a goal in patient care (Weis and others, 1983).

Many clinicians also fear that their patients will become addicted to narcotics, even though it is a rare occurrence (Porter and Jick, 1980). Marks and Sachar (1973) found that physicians prescribed even less narcotics than recommended by the literature, apparently out of fear of addiction. Nurses also tend to administer an amount in the lower dosage range of the physician's order (Cohen, 1980; Donovan, Dillon, and McGuire, 1987; Slattery, Harmer, Rosen, and Vickers, 1983; Kuhn and others, 1990), apparently for the same reason. In other studies, (Cohen, 1980; Weis and others, 1983; Charap, 1978), clinicians overestimated the risk of addiction and demonstrated a lack of knowledge about the use of analgesics. In a thoughtful editorial, Angell (1982) hypothesized that patients were undertreated because of these fears and wrote that she could not "think of any other area in medicine in which such an extravagant concern for side effects so drastically limits treatment."

Even clinicians who are skilled at assessing pain, who want their patients to be free from pain, and who are well versed in the use of narcotics may treat pain management as a secondary priority when they are preoccupied with complex biochemical and technical treatment regimens viewed as life-saving or when they are simply very busy. Treating pain in the conventional manner through the administration of narcotics by intramuscular injection on an "as needed" basis, requires clinicians to assess the level of pain a patient is experiencing at frequent intervals. Pain is not reported as a symptom on laboratory requisitions or tracked and graphically depicted on bedside vital sign charts, and it may therefore completely escape a busy clinician's attention (Max, 1990). Donovan, Dillon, and McGuire (1987) found that only 45 percent of patients who experienced pain could remember a nurse discussing it with them, and in only 49 percent of the cases were there any progress notes relating to pain in the patient's chart.

Even under the best of circumstances, the conventional approach to acute pain management results in inadequate pain relief for many patients. This approach entails the use of "prn" (*pro re nata*, as needed) orders for intramuscular narcotics. Usually, the physician specifies a dosage range and a time interval between doses, leaving the decision about the exact dosage and schedule to the judgment of the nurse. The medication the patient receives, then, is dependent on the patient's communication about the pain level and the nurse's assessment of it. The response to narcotics also varies from person to person (Tamsen, Hartvig, Fagerlund, and

Dahlström, 1982). And the delay between a patient's perception of pain and actually receiving relief may be prolonged (Vaché, 1982; Owen, McMillan, and Rogowski, 1990), given all the steps involved. These steps include summoning the nurse and having the nurse assess the pain and decide to administer medication. Then the nurse has to find the keys to the narcotics cabinet, complete the documentation required for dispensing narcotics, and actually administer the medication. For sound pharmocokinetic and logistic reasons, this approach fails to deliver complete or consistent pain relief. Instead, it results in a peak-trough cycle, in which the patients are alternately in severe pain (when they perceive the pain and complain about it) and (once the medication "kicks in") pain-free but sedated (Bauman, Gutschi, and Bivins, 1986).

Approaches to Improving Pain Management

Before they commit resources to the "problem" of pain management, hospital managers need to assess the scope of the problem in their own institution and generate the hard statistics needed to convince clinicians that it is not adequately addressed. Administrators at the University of Chicago Hospitals did not suspect a problem, for example, until they found that 86 percent of the medical and surgical patients responding to the Picker/Commonwealth survey who had pain while they were in the hospital described it as either "moderate" or "severe." An anesthesiologist at another institution trying to launch a pain control program among surgical patients found many surgeons unwilling to give up direct control of this aspect of care and reluctant to believe that their patients suffered any significant pain. Even a simple patient survey can tell clinicians and managers whether there is, indeed, a problem that needs to be addressed. The survey does not have to be elaborate, but it must solicit direct testimony from a large enough representative group of patients to be credible. A number of instruments are available for this purpose (McGuire, 1984; Acute Pain Management Guideline Panel, 1992), including the questions we developed for our telephone survey of discharged hospital patients, and visual analog devices that help hospitalized patients gauge their degree of pain.

Even asking patients to rate their pain on a scale from one to ten can be useful.

Once a problem has been identified, one of the most effective technologies developed over the past twenty years for controlling pain is patient-controlled analgesia (PCA). PCA overcomes many of the problems associated with the conventional approach by giving rational adult patients control over their own analgesia medication. The PCA device allows them to self-administer small amounts of prescribed narcotics intravenously using a control that resembles a nurse call button. They are therefore able to control the amount of pain medication they receive more precisely and consistently. The device is set in advance to control the amount of medication delivered at each push of the button, with a "lockout" interval that limits how often the button can be pushed. In theory, then, instead of riding a roller coaster between pain and grogginess, patients are able to maintain the fine balance that maximizes effective pain relief while minimizing undesirable side effects.

The theory seems to hold up in practice, according to researchers:

- While there is considerable variation in the amount of medication individual patients consume, patients tend to maintain relatively constant plasma medication levels to achieve pain relief (Tamsen and others, 1979; Tamsen, Hartvig, Fagerlund, and Dahlström, 1982; Check, 1982).
- Severe side effects, including addiction, respiratory depression, sedation, nausea, vomiting, constipation, and cough suppression, are rare (Ferrante, Orav, Rocco, and Gallo, 1988; Bauman, Gutschi, and Bivins, 1986; Keeri-Szanto, 1979; Bennett and others, 1982; Citron and others, 1986; Tamsen and others, 1979).
- Some patients require less medication than if they were treated conventionally (Sechzer, 1971; Keeri-Szanto and Heaman, 1972).
- Some researchers have also suggested that PCA may improve outcomes by sustaining more normal sleep-wake cycles, helping patients get out of bed and move around earlier after surgery, improving pulmonary functions, and thereby contributing to fewer postoperative complications (Tamsen and others, 1982; Bennett and others, 1982).

Studies of PCA have also consistently shown that patients prefer it to staff-administered medication (Kluger and Owen, 1990; Keeri-Szanto and Heaman, 1972; Raj, Knarr, Runyon, and Hopson, 1987; Bennett and others, 1982; Ferrante, Orav, Rocco, and Gallo, 1988; Citron and others, 1986; Bauman, Gutschi, and Bivins, 1986). Not only do patients report getting better and faster pain relief, they are reassured by the immediacy of relief, their control over it, and the autonomy and privacy that this control affords. Nurses have also responded well to the convenience and effectiveness of PCA, and they appreciate the time it saves them (Raj, Knarr, Runyon, and Hopson, 1987). To the extent PCA reduces postoperative complications and facilitates recovery, it may also reduce lengths of stay and hospital costs (Slack and Faut-Callahan, 1991). Anecdotal evidence suggests that physicians' acceptance of PCA is related to their experience: those who have used it like it, and those who have not may be reluctant to give up direct control of pain medication.

Successful PCA programs in hospitals have been established under the auspices of departments of anesthesia (Gilliland, 1991; Notcutt and Morgan, 1990), nursing (Hylka and Shaw, 1991; Doyle, 1991), and pharmacy (McCall and Dierks, 1990). Many programs develop uniform policies that identify factors that make patients eligible or ineligible for PCA, specify the clinicians authorized to operate and inspect the machines, and standardize orders and patient assessment procedures. Administrators who wish to implement a PCA program must also allocate time and resources for both clinician and patient education. Nurses need to learn about the technology and about the need for continuing patient assessment. Patients need to learn how to operate the machines and to understand that they cannot accidentally overdose themselves. Educational materials are often available through the companies that sell PCA devices, and many hospitals have developed their own materials (Gilliland, 1991; Hylka and Shaw, 1991).

Pain assessment must also be an ongoing part of patient care. Tracking the intensity of pain and charting it along with vital signs would make it difficult to overlook. Although busy clinicians may overlook pain control in spite of their best intentions, it is vitally important to make a baseline assessment of a patient's pain, to make regular and ongoing assessments, and to monitor the effectiveness of pain control measures as well as their side effects. Trend charting of pain status similar to conventional charting for vital signs makes these data visible and helps remind caregivers to ask patients about their level of discomfort. Asking patients to rate their pain can also help them communicate about it. Some patients deny the presence of pain until they are asked to describe it or quantify it on a scale (Donovan, Dillon, and McGuire, 1987).

Patients may also need to be educated about their right to pain relief and encouraged to take an active role in managing their pain. Patients may have misconceptions about pain and low expectations of pain relief. They may believe that pain is inevitable and untreatable, that it is somehow their own fault, that they will be seen as weak if they cannot live with it, or that they will become drug addicts if they accept medication. Although we cannot change all of the cultural factors that contribute to such views, we can take steps to help patients understand they do not need to suffer in silence. Statements about the right to pain relief might accompany the Patient's Bill of Rights that many hospitals give patients in their admitting packets. Clinicians can also raise the subject with patients, describing the discomfort they can expect and the options for dealing with it, encouraging the patient to communicate about it, and being alert to possible barriers to effective treatment. As lengths of stay become shorter, providers and patients have less time together to discuss care during the hospitalization. Some hospitals use the preadmission visit to discuss PCA or other pain control techniques with scheduled surgical patients who are to be admitted on the morning of their surgery (Doyle, 1991). Clinicians must also remember that no technology or medication substitutes for attentive patient care. Though patients like PCA, they express one reservation: that it might decrease their contact with nurses (Kluger and Owen, 1990). Pain control is not only a technical problem, nor should technical strategies be viewed as a justification for cutting staff. Central to effective pain control strategies is the caregiver's evaluation of the patient and the patient's response to treatment.

This discussion has focused on general approaches to pain control. For information on management of pain in specific types of patients or in specific medical conditions, we refer the reader to the rich literature on pain management, including the guidelines

published by the Agency for Health Care Policy and Research
(Acute Pain Management Guideline Panel, 1992).

Basic Nursing Care

The second aspect of the physical comfort dimension is basic nursing care. One physician wrote to us about his own experiences as
a patient. "What I wanted was someone with basic human kindness
who would understand the fundamental factors of fatigue, need for
sleep, personal privacy, and just being left alone from time to time."

Challenges

Under normal circumstances, most people can take care of themselves. But illness, medical treatment, and hospital confinement
create their own physical dependencies, their own discomforts. Hospital patients may need help maintaining their personal hygiene,
eating, turning over, getting up, or walking. The physical sensations and discomfort they experience are likely to be unfamiliar;
they have no way of gauging what is "normal" or expected. They
may need others to do things for them simply because they are not
familiar enough with the hospital environment to manage effectively on their own. They need timely and effective help that is
sensitive and caring. Traditionally, this basic care has been defined
as a nursing function, although the division of labor on the ward
may be such that many of the tasks are performed by other staff.
Leaving aside the technical aspects of nursing, we will focus on the
components of caring, from the patients' perspective, and on three
recurrent themes: the need for physical care, relief from discomfort,
and personal attention.

*What patients want first is attention to their basic physical
needs.* In almost any subjective hierarchy of needs, basic bodily
functions will rank first: eating, drinking, eliminating, sleeping,
moving, bathing, and grooming. Until these basic human needs are
met, individuals may not be able to move on to function or interact
at higher levels. Given their state of dependency, hospital patients
are acutely aware of these needs and how they are respected and
attended to. It is what they notice *first* about their nursing care. One

woman recalled, with gratitude, her nurse's kind assistance: "The first day I could take a shower was Saturday. I could have managed to do it myself, or I could have waited for my husband to come in, but my nurse *helped* me into the shower. I can't tell you how much that meant to me." Relying on others for their most personal care, patients are also sensitive to their caregivers' manner in tending them: "One nurse was washing me up, and oh, she was so rough!" (Riemen, 1986). Sleep is one bodily function that seems to get little attention; patients often complain of not being able to sleep in the hospital. Though environmental factors and hospital schedules must often seem to conspire to prevent sleep, patients also view their caregivers as at least partly responsible. As one particularly disgruntled patient told us: "Of all things, they would wake me up about 4:30 in the morning and get me on the scale and weigh me."

Although basic physical care rates high in importance to patients, nurses often assign it a relatively low priority in favor of technically more sophisticated or intellectually more challenging nursing functions, and some aspects of physical care may fall through the cracks. Twenty-five percent of the patients interviewed in our national survey reported being awakened sometimes or often for "no reason." A number of patients reported not getting the help they needed to go to the bathroom (7 percent) or to bathe (6 percent). Patients who failed to receive help with these most essential activities of daily living were three to four times more likely to say they would not return to the hospital in the future than those who reported no problems in these areas.

Patients rely on their caregivers to recognize and alleviate their physical discomfort. Patients notice and appreciate efforts to make them more comfortable. As one patient recalled, "One thing that made an impression on me [was that] one nurse always shaved me first before she put the tape on my arm—they should all do that." One family member described how a nurse helped an ICU patient: "They were weaning her off the ventilator, and the resident wanted to stick her arm for a blood test about every hour, and that really hurt. But the nurse took him on and said it wasn't necessary, that she would watch her closely, and finally he gave in." Patients and family members also notice caregivers' apparent insensitivity to such matters: "My father would have been so much more comfortable if they had just let him sleep on his side. And he was so thin by then. . . . Why couldn't they remember to put a pillow between his knees?"

From the point of view of these patients and their families, what mattered most was that their caregivers went out of their way (or *should* have gone out of their way) for them. They took the initiative to find a more comfortable alternative to the standard operating procedure, to tailor care to the individuals. To do so, they needed the technical competence to know when and how far they might depart from established protocols and the power and authority to negotiate with the physicians in charge on the patients' behalf. Such extra effort is not uncommon in our hospitals. Of the patients interviewed in our national survey, 82 percent reported that someone on the hospital staff went out of the way to make them feel better, and 86 percent of those identified nurses as the ones who had done so.

Effective caregivers use their knowledge and creativity to solve such problems every day. Such skilled nursing requires an understanding of the patients' coping styles and their ability to participate in their own care, and the ability to demonstrate alternatives when one approach does not work. Useful strategies for easing physical discomfort may include special positioning, application of heat or cold, immobilization, massage, breathing exercises, relaxation techniques, distraction, guided imagery, or other techniques.

Patients rely on their caregivers to be attentive and present. Asked what they look for in their nurses, patients often refer to an expert monitoring function. They want nurses to check on them frequently, to be responsive to their calls, to be prompt and efficient, and to be technically competent (Meterko, Nelson, and Rubin, 1990; Taylor, Hudson, and Keeling, 1991; Larson, 1984; Cronin and Harrison, 1988; Riemen, 1986; Tagliacozzo, 1965). Patients are reassured knowing not just that help is available if they need it, but that concerned professionals are monitoring them and their care. As one patient told us, "The nurse came in and asked if there was anything I wanted and how did I feel. I know it sounds inconsequential, but that made me feel so good, like if there was anything I ever needed, it would be there."

And one of the most frustrating experiences for a helpless hospital patient is to have *no one* available. Twenty-eight percent of patients interviewed in our national survey said their nurses at some time seemed "too busy" to take care of them, and 77 percent of those said this happened more than once. Those who found this often to be the case were nearly six times as likely to say they would never return to the hospital again. Five percent of the hospital patients we surveyed also reported waiting more than fifteen minutes, on average, to have their call buttons answered. These patients were more than four times more likely than other patients surveyed to say they would never return.

Besides being available, patients need nurses and other caregivers to be mentally present and approachable. Many patients cite attributes among nursing staff such as having a pleasant personality, being courteous, acting in a "professional" manner, and being accessible as important (Tagliacozzo, 1965; Henry, 1975; Press, Ganey, and Malone, 1991; Larson, 1984). On the other hand, patients identified behaviors such as being in a hurry, doing only what has to be done, and approaching their work as "just a job" where nothing really matters as evidence that caregivers did not really care (Rieman, 1986).

Being truly "present" requires perceptive communication and genuine empathy. The French philosopher Marcel described such presence: "It is an undeniable fact [that] there are some people who reveal themselves as 'present'—that is to say, at our disposal— when we are in pain or need to confide in someone, while there are other people who do not give this feeling, however great is their goodwill. . . . The most attentive listener may give me the impression of not being present; he gives me nothing, he cannot make room for me in himself whatever the material favors he is prepared to grant me. The truth is, there is a way of listening which is a way of giving, and another way which is a way of refusing. . . . Presence is something which reveals itself immediately and unmistakably in a look, a smile, an intonation, or a handshake" (quoted in Riemen, 1986, p. 35).

Are our patients this perceptive? Yes! Presence entails the capacity to listen, to be perceptive to the environment, and to anticipate a patient's needs.

Solutions

What can hospitals do to enhance the quality of basic nursing care? Above all, as we stress throughout this book, they need to understand what patients experience while they are in the hospital and how they perceive their basic care. This entails soliciting input from patients on a regular and routine basis, through surveys, focus groups, and other devices. Only in this way can staff begin to understand their work from the patient's perspective and identify strong and weak points in their performance on the job. Hearing patients report firsthand about their care is the most compelling and constructive form of criticism. Surveys at the nursing unit level can give unit staff structured feedback about how they are doing compared to others in the hospital and reinforce the progress they make over time.

Caregivers should also make expectations about basic care explicit. Although it may seem obvious to most clinicians that patients should get whatever help or special assistance they need to get better, the importance of basic physical care may be so obvious that no one really thinks about it. Hospital or nursing unit "culture" cannot be relied on to transmit expectations about patient care. All unit staff need to review procedures together to define the components of basic care, identify the appropriate caregiver, and make explicit the standards of behavior that staff will be expected to observe. Topics for discussion and standard setting might include how best to provide timely assistance for patients requesting it; offering help with bathing or eating (and when it is appropriate to encourage patients' independence in those tasks); staff behavior at night; the appropriateness of discussing personal matters in front of patients; and such courtesies as knocking on doors, offering a choice of times for baths and treatments, or volunteering to return later when a family member is present. Developing more patient-centered approaches may also entail enlisting the cooperation of professional and nonprofessional workers who report outside the nursing unit, including physicians, transport workers, housekeeping staff, technicians, phlebotomists, and therapists.

Supervisors must find appropriate ways to review and reinforce the standards on a continuing basis, to monitor staff performance, and to provide incentives for good care. Staff at all levels who provide excellent basic care should be recognized for their contributions to patient comfort. They should be rewarded for their creativity, their interaction with patients, and their sensitivity to basic physical needs as well as for their technical proficiency. When patient feedback demonstrates improvement, staff efforts should be recognized and reinforced. By the same token, staff who cannot or will not meet explicit standards of care should be reassigned to non–patient care areas. Recognizing and rewarding patient-centered care may require managers and staff to change their perspective. Hospital workers, including nursing staff, work for the approval of their supervisors and co-workers as much as they work for patients. In such an atmosphere, the nurse who wakes patients up in the wee hours of the morning to remake their beds, "freshen them up," and tidy their rooms before the next shift arrives is likely to be popular among her co-workers. But this is hardly *patient*-centered care; it is *nurse*-centered care.

Hospitals also need to seek ways to maximize the time nursing staff have to spend with patients and to care for them. Are those charged with patient care performing noncare tasks others could do? Can work be reorganized or physically rearranged to make it more efficient? Can charting and other nursing paperwork be made simpler, faster? Keeping often-used supplies in patients' rooms, for example, can save time. Placing computer terminals in patients' rooms, where nursing staff can check records and complete most documentation, similarly reduces the amount of time spent in the nursing station to perform such tasks. New electronic communication systems can reduce the time it takes to answer call buttons and track down the appropriate caregiver. Enlisting the help of families and friends in caring for patients and allowing patients, families, and visitors to help themselves to commonly needed supplies can also free staff time for other caregiving functions.

The Physical Environment

Our final topic related to physical comfort is the hospital itself. As one patient observed, "When you're really terribly physically sick, you want your life saved. When you're feeling better, you start caring about what your environment looks like."

We all recognize the effect our physical surroundings have on us. Who has not luxuriated in the warmth of the sun on a perfect day, or reveled in the hug of an overstuffed chair while reading a favorite book? And who has not squirmed in the suffocating embrace of a too-hot, too-humid day, or given up on accomplishing a mental task in the midst of jarring construction noise outside the window? We perceive our physical surroundings as being comforting or hostile based on our five senses. And sometimes a "sixth sense" hints at things we cannot observe directly. Although patients in our focus groups often spoke prominently about the hospital's physical environment, our national survey focused mostly on the interpersonal aspects of care, and the reader will note the absence of survey data in this section. Nevertheless, patients *do* notice the hospital itself, and keeping their perceptions in mind when redesigning space can enhance patient-centered care. Here, we first consider how the environment affects well-being. We then turn our attention to the specific aspects of the hospital environment most important to patients and their families.

A Healing Environment

Our perception of our surroundings affects our mood and thinking in ways we may not recognize. In one interesting study, Maslow and Mintz (1956) experimented with the effect of aesthetic surroundings on people by seating subjects in three different rooms, described as "beautiful," "average," and "ugly." The "beautiful" room contained a soft armchair, window drapes, pictures, and a colorful rug. The "ugly" room contained a small table, straight-backed chairs, full ashtrays, and assorted refuse. The "average" room had gray walls, a mahogany desk, a metal filing cabinet, and other features that made it look like a worked-in office. The subjects were asked to rate the energy and well-being of faces in photographs, but they were not told about the real purpose of the experiment. Although the subjects were shown identical photographs, those seated in the "beautiful" room gave them ratings that were significantly higher on the energy/well-being scale. Ratings were lower in the "average" room and lower still in the "ugly" room.

In a more recent study, Chaikin, Derlega, and Miller (1976) interviewed subjects in two different rooms designed to represent "soft" and "hard" architecture. A small, windowless room with an asphalt tile floor, cinderblock walls, and overhead fluorescent light was left in its original "hard" condition for one group of interviews; it was furnished with "soft" features such as an oriental rug, cushioned armchair, and magazines for another group. The investigators found that subjects were willing to disclose more intimate information and appeared to feel more relaxed in the "soft" room than the "hard" one. Still other studies have shown that air quality, noise, and privacy are strong predictors of psychological well-being in a group of office workers (Klitzman and Stellman, 1989), and that "deinstitutionalizing" a hospital's appearance through the use of color and pleasant furnishings can result in more active elderly and mental patients and happier staff (Christenfeld, Wagner, Pastva, and Acrish, 1989; Cooper, Mohide, and Gilbert, 1989; Minde, Haynes, and Rodenburg, 1990; Sommer and Ross, 1958).

As patients and visitors to hospitals, our perceptions are complicated by our lack of familiarity with the surroundings and the stresses of illness and uncertainty. Just when we are least able to adapt, we are expected to adjust to unfamiliar spaces, communal living, and the rhythms of institutional life, in addition to the loss of physical privacy. We give up control of our personal lives and eat, sleep, bathe, submit to procedures, and interact with staff on the hospital's schedule, not our own.

In the past, healers have recognized the importance of comfortable, supportive surroundings, as illustrated by the European spa tradition. But modern medical practice has created hospitals designed to accommodate technology, optimize efficiency, and maintain an aseptic environment. The patient's view has rarely been considered. In the worst of these designs, patients are met by clean lines, featureless walls, and hard and shiny surfaces, all intended to be easily maintained. Soft, humanizing touches are considered luxuries. Such "hard architecture" feels unyielding and resists efforts to personalize space, increasing patients' sense of loss of control (Sommer, 1974). It has a similar effect on staff, making them uncomfortable and perhaps compromising the quality of the care they deliver (Keep, 1977). In recent years, both hospital designers and health care providers have become more conscious of the importance of physical environment to the healing process and of the need to temper hard institutional structures with softening effects that promote psychological well-being. A supportive environment may serve both the primary function of helping to prevent illness and the secondary therapeutic function of alleviating stress and depression (Winkel and Holahan, 1985). While the hospital can never be "home" to patients, the new effort is to convey a message of warmth and well-being rather than of sterility and efficiency.

What Can Hospitals Do?

Hospital managers cannot, by magic, make large, shiny, and frightening medical equipment disappear, nor can they replace existing hospital plants with beautiful new buildings. However, health care providers, researchers, and designers have developed strategies, ranging from the modest to the ambitious, that can help humanize the physical hospital environment.

Patients and staff who use and work in an area need to take part in the process of finding solutions to problems of environmental design. Bellevue Hospital in New York found that such a participatory approach offers three benefits: it minimizes the need for costly redesign of spaces that do not work, from the patients' or the staff's perspective; it boosts morale; and it conveys the message that the hospital cares about its patients and staff and values their opinions. Bellevue also made use of expert volunteers from the local community—faculty and doctoral students from the City University of New York and students from other local design schools (Bohman, 1984). Building a life-sized mock-up of a proposed design and having staff and patients walk through and use it is a good way to test it in advance.

Not surprisingly, cleanliness was the aspect of the environment that patients mentioned most prominently in our focus groups. Even though they appreciate the fact that workers may be busy, the presence of used bandages, piles of dirty laundry, or other visible "dirt" seems incongruous to them in a hospital environ-

ment, if not downright disconcerting. Even the most unsophisticated patient recognizes the relationship between cleanliness and
health, and patients see neglect of this basic principle as a major
failure.

What follows are selected suggestions relating to other aspects of the hospital environment that patients mentioned. Most of
them can be incorporated into existing structures, though some
would entail new construction. For more detailed discussion of design alternatives, we refer readers to the literature on patient-
centered hospital design (see, for example, Carpman, Grant, and
Simmons, 1986).

Create a Comfortable Hospital Environment. People need variety
and change in their sensory environment, but not so much that it
produces sensory overload. Nature should be incorporated into the
hospital environment as much as possible through the use of windows, skylights, indoor plants, running water, and landscaping that
is viewable from the interior. Natural sunlight imparts a feeling of
a healthy environment, and natural settings are soothing because of
their infinite and subtle variations. In urban settings, even a small
park can provide a place for patients, visitors, and staff to revitalize
outside the hospital.

Hospitals can also create a more pleasing interior atmosphere by incorporating different colors and textures into existing
spaces, consistent with their use and function. Some suggestions
follow:

• Works of art, especially representational treatments of natural
  subjects, can promote enjoyment and relaxation. Patients tend
  to prefer rural or wilderness landscapes that include animals,
  water, valleys, mountains, and farmland over interior or urban
  scenes or abstractions. They also prefer pictures that are textur-
  ally complex over posters with words (Carpman, Grant, and
  Simmons, 1986).
• Natural lighting should be used wherever possible. Where artificial lighting is necessary, designers and planners should bear
  in mind that nonvariable lighting tends to create an institutional atmosphere (Stone, Stone, and Giffin, 1990). Moreover,

incandescent lighting is more pleasing to patients, while fluorescent lighting casts an indiscriminate glare.

- Carpeting is perceived to be softer and "warmer" than hard floor coverings. It also helps muffle noise and provides surer footing than either linoleum or ceramic tile.

- Fabric wall coverings make rooms quieter and "warmer." Some varieties can be washed with bleach without affecting color (Birdsong and Leibrock, 1990).

- Upholstery fabric can be coated for protection. It does not need to be covered in vinyl for easy maintenance.

- Wood surfaces have a warmer feel than metal, plastic, or painted surfaces, and wood retains its character in spite of wear and tear.

- Although white surfaces may be preferred in examining rooms because they provide optimal light, they should be used sparingly in patient areas because of their glare (Birren, 1979).

- Shades of red, yellow, and orange make rooms appear warmer and more active, while "cooler" shades of blue or green make them seem more soothing and relaxing. Washed-out pastels and muddy grays, greens, and browns impart an institutional feel.

- The aging lens may be unable to distinguish among shades of blue-green, blue, and violet, but the elderly generally retain the ability to differentiate among warm colors.

- Abandoning the use of overhead speakers for paging, in favor of newer beeper and telephone technologies, helps reduce the ambient noise level.

- Using bells or other musical sounds for alarms makes them quieter and less frightening.

The Patient's Room. Patients spend most of their time in one room. It is their bedroom, living room, dining room, and maybe their bathroom. Not surprisingly, it was their rooms that our focus-group patients and their family members had most to say about. Some complained about the temperature: "I always remember being freezing in the hospital. You're sick, your body's colder—and they give you this skinny little blanket."

One family member complained about logistical problems making a patient's stay difficult: "He was put in with a very sick gentleman. And he couldn't use the bathroom facilities, because the man was near the bathroom and always had the curtain closed. You had to go through all this paraphernalia to get in. So he had to go down to one of the empty rooms." Cramped quarters were a problem: "The shower? Barely room to turn around, no place to hang your clothes, nothing."

Patients' rooms should be designed to be private spaces, free from unwanted distractions. Not all patients want a private room, however. Nearly half of the patients queried in one study preferred semiprivate rooms (Carpman, Grant, and Simmons, 1986). In another, many preferred four-bed units to private rooms (Thompson, 1955). Nevertheless, patients do want privacy, in the sense that they do not want to be viewed by everyone passing by. If possible, planners should arrange beds so that patients' feet are closest to the door.

One of the most essential features of any patient room is a window to the outdoors. Windows relieve the sense of enclosure, provide a source of natural light, help maintain circadian rhythms, and make patients feel less cut off from the outside world. Rooms should be designed and arranged so that all patients can easily look out, with beds positioned so the window is at the patients' side rather than behind their head. Views of natural landscapes are, of course, preferable wherever possible. In one study of surgical patients, Ulrich (1984) compared patients who had a view of trees with a second group that could look out only on a brick wall. He found that those who had the tree view required milder doses of analgesics, had shorter postoperative lengths of stay, experienced fewer negative comments from the nursing staff, and had slightly fewer postsurgical complications than the brick-wall group.

Some other ideas for making rooms more patient centered follow:

- A curtained window onto the corridor can make patients in private rooms feel less isolated and gives them the option of watching activity outside the room if they so desire.
- While fluorescent lights may be necessary, rooms should also have at least some incandescent lighting, and all lights should be controllable from the bed. Night lights make it easier and safer for patients to navigate to the bathroom or to the door.

- Equipment and supplies can be frightening or disconcerting and should be concealed in closets or cupboards.
- To the extent possible, painful or invasive procedures should be conducted in areas other than the patient's room.
- Patient rooms equipped with shelf space and bulletin boards permit patients to personalize their space by displaying books or other objects from home.
- Patients need ample closet space for their personal belongings, preferably with a lock and supplied with hooks as well as hangers.
- Room furnishings might include items that visiting friends or family members can convert to a bed, when necessary. Alternatively, rollout beds or cots might be kept in lounge areas or elsewhere on the unit.
- Patients find lever-type handles on doors and cabinets easier to grip than knobs.
- Headphones or pillow speakers for televisions, especially in nonprivate rooms, lower noise levels and enhance privacy.
- Movies that patients can play on VCRs in their rooms can distract them and help time pass more quickly.
- Calendars and clocks in patient rooms help keep patients oriented, but they should not be placed prominently in their line of vision.
- A rocking chair, a table or desk, or seating next to a window suggest the comforts of home. Where room allows, a table and extra chairs give patients the option of dining out of bed, possibly with visitors.
- Displaying the patient's name above the head of the bed makes it easier for all staff to remember to use the name.
- While many hospitals have relaxed their policies regarding uniforms for hospital personnel, most still require patients to wear hospital-issued gowns. Permitting patients to wear their own lounging clothes helps them retain their personal identity in an unfamiliar and impersonal environment (Giloth, 1990).

Intensive Care Units. Patients in ICUs face a particularly harsh environment. Often immobilized by pain and tubing, disoriented due to their illness or medication, and subjected to constant observation by others and total loss of privacy, their fragile sense of hope is further assaulted by bright lights, noisy machines, and a view of other critically ill patients. Patients speak of "not being able to escape," of "being tied down," or of feeling a "general sense of urgency" in the environment and a "constant threat of death" (De-Meyer, 1967). Such stress threatens not only the patients' mental well-being, but their physical recovery, if it becomes impossible for them to cooperate in therapeutic tasks such as weaning from a ventilator. Some suggestions for making the ICU less stressful follow:

- Intensive care units should have windows, and patients should be able to see outside if possible. The presence of windows and interesting views has been linked with patients' well-being (Keep, 1977; Ulrich, 1984).
- Beds should be placed in single or double rooms rather than in an open ward. In open units, consider installing partitions to separate beds visually and acoustically.
- Reduce the ambient noise by muffling telephones, turning down the volume on monitors, replacing grating alarms with musical tones, using monitors and other machines only when necessary, and turning off machines not in use. Carpets and draperies can be used to absorb sound, and the nursing station and utility area should be well insulated to reduce sound transmission.
- Reduce noise near the patient's ears by placing monitors, pumps, or other machines as far as possible from the head of the bed. Turn outflow valves and alarms away from the patient's head (Baker, 1984).
- Help patients stay oriented by placing a clock and calendar where they can see them and by dimming the lights at night.
- Place equipment outside the patients' view as much as possible. Turn monitor screens so they cannot be watched by other patients.

Visitor Waiting Areas. No matter what the patient's medical condition, nearly all visiting family members and friends spend some time in waiting areas. Some are just passing time while the patient gets ready for visitors; others are anxiously waiting for a procedure to be over and possibly fearing the arrival of bad news. The physical environment affects how people in waiting spaces feel and behave. In their classic study, Sommer and Ross (1958) described a chronic geriatric ward dayroom, in which chairs were lined up neatly against the walls, as a place where patients sat silently waiting "for a train that never comes." After rearranging the chairs in groups around tables and adding magazines and flowers, they noted a dramatic increase in patients' verbal interactions, and visitors commented on the lively new tone.

Waiting areas are no longer so stark, and many provide distractions such as television. Yet, as family members told us, certain factors can alleviate or intensify stress:

"You're staring at the pictures, waiting and waiting while they're downstairs for the angioplasty, or in the ICU, or whatever they're doing. And you just look—there's no one else in the room maybe but yourself—and you stare. And this stupid television is bouncing up and down."

"There were morbid pictures on the wall. They should have soothing, cheerful pictures."

"There was a general waiting room for families and then there was a conference room so you could have a private conversation. There were telephones that were right there available to the families, and that was very important."

Some suggestions for making waiting areas more comfortable and amenable to visitors follow:

- Waiting rooms should be arranged to allow occupants to pursue different activities, such as conversing, watching television, reading, or napping. Separate spaces can be created through thoughtful placement of the television, plants (*healthy* ones, not sick or dying ones), room dividers, and reading materials.
- Telephones should be readily accessible to visitors, in spaces that afford them acoustic privacy.
- Soft colors and lighting, plants, and aquariums help create a soothing environment. Windows and calming pictures create visual interest.
- Chairs and sofas should be grouped to accommodate varying

numbers of people. Movable tables, chairs, and sofas will help visitors create their own space.

- Frail or elderly visitors may have trouble getting up from some chairs and sofas. Seating should be selected accordingly.
- Providing family members with beepers while they are waiting for a patient undergoing a lengthy procedure minimizes the time they spend in waiting areas. Beth Israel Hospital in Boston uses beepers for families of surgical patients, so that they can leave the hospital until the doctor or patient can see them.

Diagnostic and Treatment Areas. Diagnostic procedures may be frightening in and of themselves. The patient's discomfort may also be intensified by the physical setting, as one patient eloquently described: "I had to go to radiology and angioplasty. It looks like they're taking you to the morgue. The angioplasty room . . . looks like your last stop before hell, dismal and dark. The room looks like the way you feel. That and radiology, with the bright lights and the instruments. . . . There's got to be something more conducive to making you feel this isn't the last mile." Another patient described her experience at an otherwise renowned hospital mammography unit: "After we had our mammograms, we were told to go back to the waiting room, where they would call us in with the results. We all sat there in our gowns, scared, and one by one they'd call us back in. Some women would come back out crying miserably; some would be smiling. It was awful. You just sat there wondering which you'd be." Many, many patients pass through radiology, nuclear medicine, cardiac catheterization laboratories, bronchoscopy suites, and the like. The image of an assembly line often comes to mind. Patients arrive at the area and see other apprehensive patients, spend some time waiting for a technician or equipment before the procedure gets under way, assume an uncomfortable position against one or more hard surfaces, then submit to a procedure that most likely involves mechanical devices, discomfort, and deep invasion of body privacy. While there is no substitute for emotional support, information, and the appropriate use of pain and tranquilizing medications, these technical areas can also be humanized in their physical design and arrangement. Some suggestions follow.

- Natural scenes, mobiles, or other relaxing images placed in the patient's line of sight provide distraction. If the patient must be supine for the procedure, pictures might be placed on the ceiling (Oberlander, 1979).

- The "high-tech" feeling of a room can be alleviated with soft colors and lighting and textured floor and wall coverings. Large, shiny equipment should be concealed or made less imposing by painting it the same color as the walls.

- Whenever it is technically feasible, patients' physical contact with cold metal equipment should be minimized or softened with the use of blankets and pillows.

- People tend to feel exposed and vulnerable when they are placed in the middle of a room. Patients will find it more comfortable to have their backs to the wall, where they can see what is going on around them, and to be approached from the front.

- The room temperature should be warm enough for patients dressed in simple cotton gowns.

- When procedures do not require patients' active cooperation, listening to a variety (or a choice) of music through stereo headsets or pillow speakers is comforting and distracting.

- Space should be arranged to route traffic so that patients do not have to be scrutinized by others. Seeing other sick patients in varying physical and emotional states on their way to or from a procedure can be frightening and upsetting (Kimball, 1984).

- Waiting patients should be approached personally, when it is their turn for a procedure, rather than called from across the room or over a loudspeaker. Asking ambulatory patients to sit in color-coded (or otherwise distinguishable) chairs can help receptionists identify them.

Corridors. Hospital corridors are often quite long and tend to be designed for efficiency of transportation rather than the comfort of those passing through. A clean and shiny hallway may look sterile and impersonal, from the perspective of patients and visitors, and may create an emotional obstacle to entering (Shield, 1990). Furthermore, corridors that are long, featureless, and poorly lit can seem intimidating and may be a source of disturbing visual and auditory distortions (Spivak, 1967). Corridors can be made more inviting in a number of ways:

- When buildings are designed, corridors might be placed along outside walls, adjacent to scenic areas that can be viewed through windows along the way. However, windows should not be placed at the ends of long, straight, and otherwise windowless hallways.
- Reflection and glare can be reduced through the use of dense, low-pile carpeting (that carts and gurneys can roll over) and nonreflective wall and ceiling coverings, and by breaking up long, shiny surfaces.
- Lubricating wheels or using rubber wheels on carts and gurneys reduces noise, as they are rolled through corridors.
- Photographs of outdoor scenes, murals, textile pieces, and paintings add interest and texture to walls. Painted murals, mobiles, or other artworks on the ceiling give patients traveling by gurney something interesting to look at.
- Periodic overhead lighting produces glare and shines in the eyes of patients on gurneys. Continuous low-intensity lighting along one wall is preferable.
- Handrails should be mounted on both sides of the corridor.
- Placing room entrances so that they are not directly across the hall from one another helps keep noise from traveling from one room to another. Indenting doors to create a vestibule-like entry also breaks up the long lines of a corridor and helps create a transition area to the room.
- Maps and signs should be simple and easy to read. Maps should be oriented in the direction readers are facing so they do not have to "turn around" mentally to find their way.
- Wherever possible, separate elevators should be provided for patients, visitors, and service staff.

Summary

We have considered three aspects of physical comfort that patients tell us are important to them: pain control, basic nursing care, and the hospital's physical environment. Each deserves attention from caregivers, including thought about ways of soliciting patients' feedback about them. Hospitals need to use this information to develop strategies to improve physical care. Physical comfort is the most basic service hospitals offer patients, and it is a sick person's most fundamental right.

The management of pain is complex. Pain control is affected by the attitudes of patients and clinicians and the quality of communication between them, and by individuals' different responses to therapy. Patient-controlled analgesia is an effective technology for managing pain that has proved to be popular with both patients and clinicians. Other important strategies involve making pain assessment data more visible to caregivers and raising patients' expectations about pain relief.

Patients are acutely aware of their dependency on others to take care of their most basic physical needs, and they are more likely not to return to hospitals that fail to meet those needs. Unfortunately, basic physical care is often taken for granted and is therefore rarely addressed explicitly. Nurses and other caregivers need to define care standards and reward the delivery of outstanding basic care. New technologies may also offer ways to free nurses and others from noncare activities, enabling them to spend more time with patients.

And finally, a patient's experience of illness can be seriously affected by the physical environment of the hospital—its unfamiliarity, its institutional character, its frightening sights and sounds. Although not every aspect of the physical plant and equipment of a medical care facility will be amenable to change, sensitivity to patients' perceptions and experiences can make it a more humane environment. Above all, patients need to be involved both in identifying problems and, together with the staff who work there, in helping designers find solutions.

Suggestions for Improvement

- To help patients communicate about their pain, ask them to rate it on a scale of one to ten.
- Do trend charting of patients' pain status on their bedside vital signs sheets.

- Make pain relief part of the Patient's Bill of Rights.
- Introduce or expand the use of patient-controlled analgesia.
- Run a seminar for all clinical staff on your institution's current pain control protocols. Include discussion of misconceptions about narcotics and their true risks and benefits.
- Create avenues for rewarding excellent basic nursing care. Recognize nurses or other staff singled out by patients, families, or peers.
- To the extent possible, schedule routine procedures such as blood drawing, bathing, weighing, and daily x-rays around patients' normal sleep cycles.
- Use natural and incandescent lighting wherever possible.
- Provide shelf space and bulletin boards in patients' rooms to permit them to personalize their space by displaying cards or objects from home.
- Equip waiting areas with movable tables, chairs, and sofas to allow visitors to create their own space.

References

Acute Pain Management Guideline Panel. *Acute Pain Management: Operative or Medical Procedures and Trauma: Clinical Practice Guideline.* AHCPR Publication No. 92-0032. Rockville, Md.: Agency for Health Care Policy and Research, Public Health Service, U.S. Department of Health and Human Services, 1992.

Angell, M. "The Quality of Mercy." *New England Journal of Medicine,* 1982, *306,* 98–99.

Baer, E., Davitz, L. J., and Lieb, R. "Inferences of Physical Pain and Psychological Distress. 1: In Relation to Verbal and Nonverbal Patient Communication." *Nursing Research,* 1970, *19,* 83–92.

Baker, C. F. "Sensory Overload and Noise in the ICU: Sources of Environmental Stress." *Critical Care Quarterly,* 1984, *6,* 66–80.

Bauman, T. J., Gutschi, L. M., and Bivins, B. A. "The Safety and Efficacy of a New Patient-Controlled Analgesia Device in Hospitalized Trauma and Surgery Patients." *Henry Ford Hospital Medical Journal,* 1986, *34,* 105–108.

Beecher, H. K. "Relationship of Significance of Wound to Pain

Experienced." *Journal of the American Medical Association,* 1956, *161,* 1609–1613.

Bennett, R. L., and others. "Patient-Controlled Analgesia: A New Concept of Postoperative Pain Relief." *Annals of Surgery,* 1982, *195,* 700–705.

Birdsong, C., and Leibrock, C. "Patient-Centered Design." *Healthcare Forum Journal,* 1990, *33,* 40–45.

Birren, F. "Human Response to Color and Light." *Hospitals,* July 16, 1979, pp. 93–96.

Bohman, M. A. "Environmental Design Boosts Patient, Staff Morale." *Hospital Manager,* 1984, *14,* 5–6.

Carpman, J. R., Grant, M. A., and Simmons, D. A. *Design That Cares: Planning Health Facilities for Patients and Visitors.* Chicago: American Hospital Publishing, 1986.

Chaikin, A. L., Derlega, V. J., and Miller, S. J. "Effects of Room Environment on Self-Disclosure in a Counseling Analogue." *Journal of Counseling and Psychology,* 1976, *23,* 479–481.

Charap, A. D. "The Knowledge, Attitudes, and Experience of Medical Personnel Treating Pain in the Terminally Ill." *Mt. Sinai Journal of Medicine (New York),* 1978, *45,* 561–580.

Check, W. A. "Results Are Better When Patients Control Their Own Analgesia." *Journal of the American Medical Association,* 1982, *247,* 945–947.

Christenfeld, R., Wagner, J., Pastva, G., and Acrish, W. P. "How Physical Settings Affect Chronic Mental Patients." *Psychology Quarterly,* 1989, *60,* 253–264.

Citron, M. L., and others. "Patient-Controlled Analgesia for Severe Cancer Pain." *Archives of Internal Medicine,* 1986, *146,* 734–736.

Cohen, F. L. "Postsurgical Pain Relief: Patients' Status and Nurses' Medication Choices." *Pain,* 1980, *9,* 265–274.

Cooper, B., Mohide, A., and Gilbert, S. "Testing the Use of Color in a Long-Term Care Setting." *Dimensions,* 1989, *66,* 22–26.

Cronin, S. N., and Harrison, B. "Importance of Nurse Caring Behaviors as Perceived by Patients After Myocardial Infarction." *Heart & Lung,* 1988, *17*(4), 374–380.

DeMeyer, J. "The Environment of the Intensive Care Unit." *Nursing Forum,* 1967, *6,* 262–272.

Diers, D., Schmidt, R. L., McBride, M.A.B., and Davis, B. L. "The

Effect of Nursing Interaction on Patients in Pain." *Nursing Research*, 1972, *21*, 419–428.

Donovan, B. D. "Patient Attitudes to Postoperative Pain Relief." *Anesthesia and Intensive Care*, 1983, *11*, 125–129.

Donovan, M., Dillon, P., and McGuire, L. "Incidence and Characteristics of Pain in a Sample of Medical-Surgical Inpatients." *Pain*, 1987, *30*, 69–78.

Doyle, L. "Patient-Controlled Analgesia in the Postanesthesia Care Unit: One Unit's Approach." *Journal of Post Anesthesia Nursing*, 1991, *6*(2), 93–97.

Egbert, L. D., Battit, G. E., Welch, C. E., and Bartlett, M. K. "Reduction of Postoperative Pain by Encouragement and Instruction of Patients: A Study of Doctor-Patient Rapport." *New England Journal of Medicine*, 1964, *270*, 825–827.

Ferrante, F. M., Orav, E. J., Rocco, A. G., and Gallo, J. "A Statistical Model for Pain in Patient-Controlled Analgesia and Conventional Intramuscular Opioid Regimens." *Anesthesia and Analgesia*, 1988, *67*, 457–461.

Gilliland, C. L. "Patient-Controlled Analgesia: A New Method for Pain Control." *Comprehensive Therapy*, 1991, *17*(1), 34–41.

Giloth, B. E. "Promoting Patient Involvement: Educational, Organizational, and Environmental Strategies." *Patient Education and Counseling*, 1990, *15*, 29–38.

Graffam, S. "Congruence of Nurse-Patient Expectations Regarding Nursing Intervention in Pain." *Nursing Leadership*, 1981, *4*(2), 12–15.

Henry, O.M.M. "Nurse Behaviors Perceived by Patients as Indicators of Caring." Unpublished doctoral dissertation, Department of Nursing, the Catholic University of America. *Dissertation Abstracts International*, *36*, 02652B, 1975.

Hylka, S. C., and Shaw, C. F. "Implementation of a Patient-Controlled Analgesia Program Under the Direction of the Nursing Department." *Journal of Post Anesthesia Nursing*, 1991, *6*(3), 170–175.

Keep, P. J. "Stimulus Deprivation in Windowless Rooms." *Anaesthesia*, 1977, *32*(7), 598–602.

Keeri-Szanto, M. "Drugs or Drums: What Relieves Postoperative Pain?" *Pain*, 1979, *6*, 217–230.

Keeri-Szanto, M., and Heaman, S. "Postoperative Demand Analgesia." *Surgical Gynecology and Obstetrics*, 1972, *134*, 647–651.

Kimball, E. "Interior Design as Healing Agent." *Canadian Medical Association Journal*, 1984, *130*, 1364–1372.

Klitzman, S., and Stellman, J. M. "The Impact of the Physical Environment on the Psychological Well-Being of Office Workers." *Social Science in Medicine*, 1989, *29*, 733–742.

Kluger, M. T., and Owen, H. "Forum: Patients' Expectations of Patient-Controlled Analgesia." *Anaesthesia*, 1990, *45*, 1072–1074.

Kuhn, S., and others. "Perceptions of Pain Relief after Surgery." *British Medical Journal*, 1990, *300*, 1687–1690.

Larson, P. "Important Nurse Caring Behaviors Perceived by Patients with Cancer." *Oncology Nursing Forum*, 1984, *11*(6), 46–50.

Larson, P. "Comparison of Cancer Patients' and Professional Nurses' Perceptions of Important Nurse Caring Behaviors." *Heart & Lung*, 1987, *16*(2), 187–193.

Lim, A. T., and others. "Postoperative Pain Control: Contribution of Psychological Factors and Transcutaneous Electrical Stimulation." *Pain*, 1983, *17*, 179–188.

McCall, L. J., and Dierks, D. R. "Pharmacy-Managed Patient-Controlled Analgesia Service." *American Journal of Hospital Pharmacy*, 1990, *47*, 2706–2710.

McGuire, D. B. "The Measurement of Clinical Pain." *Nursing Research*, 1984, *33*, 152–156.

Marks, R. M., and Sachar, E. J. "Undertreatment of Medical Inpatients with Narcotic Analgesics." *Annals of Internal Medicine*, 1973, *78*, 173–181.

Maslow, A. H., and Mintz, N. L. "Effects of Esthetic Surroundings. 1: Initial Effects of Three Esthetic Conditions upon Perceiving 'Energy' and 'Well-Being' in Faces." *Journal of Psychology*, 1956, *41*, 247–254.

Max, M. B. "Improving Outcomes of Analgesic Treatment: Is Education Enough?" *Annals of Internal Medicine*, 1990, *113*, 885–889.

Meterko, M., Nelson, E. C., and Rubin, H. R. "Patient Judgments of Hospital Quality: Report of a Pilot Study." *Medical Care*, 1990 Supplement, *28*(9), S1–S56.

Minde, R., Haynes, E., and Rodenburg, M. "The Ward Milieu and Its Effect on the Behavior of Psychogeriatric Patients." *Canadian Journal of Psychology*, 1990, *35*, 133–138.

Notcutt, W. G., and Morgan, R.J.M. "Introducing Patient-Controlled Analgesia for Postoperative Pain Control into a District General Hospital." *Anaesthesia*, 1990, *45*, 401–406.

Oberlander, R. "Beauty in a Hospital Aids the Cure." *Hospitals*, 1979, *53*, 89–92.

Owen, H., McMillan, V., and Rogowski, D. "Postoperative Pain Therapy: A Survey of Patients' Expectations and Their Experiences." *Pain*, 1990, *41*, 303–307.

Pernick, M. S. "The Calculus of Suffering in Nineteenth Century Surgery." *Hastings Center Report*, 1983, *13*, 26–36.

Porter, J., and Jick, H. "Addiction Rare in Patients Treated with Narcotics." *New England Journal of Medicine*, 1980, *302*, 123.

Press, I., Ganey, R. F., and Malone, M. P. "Satisfied Patients Can Spell Financial Well-Being." *Healthcare Financial Management*, 1991, *45*(2), 34–40.

Puntillo, K. A. "Pain Experiences of Intensive Care Unit Patients." *Heart & Lung*, 1990, *19*(5, part 1), 526–533.

Raj, P. R., Knarr, D., Runyon, J., and Hopson, C. N. "Patient-Controlled Analgesia for Postoperative Pain in Orthopaedic Patients." *Orthopedics Review*, 1987, *16*, 953–959.

Rankin, M. A., and Snider, B. "Nurses' Perceptions of Cancer Patients' Pain." *Cancer Nursing*, 1984, *7*, 149–155.

Riemen, D. J. "Noncaring and Caring in the Clinical Setting: Patients' Descriptions." *Topics in Clinical Nursing*, 1986, *8*(2), 30–36.

Sechzer, P. H. "Studies in Pain with the Analgesic-Demand System." *Anesthesia and Analgesia Current Research*, 1971, *50*, 1–10.

Shield, R. R. "Pathways and Porches: A Focus on Corridors in Nursing Homes." *Rhode Island Medical Journal*, 1990, *73*, 155–160.

Slack, J., and Faut-Callahan, M. "Pain Management." *Nursing Clinics of North America*, 1991, *26*, 463–476.

Slattery, P. J., Harmer, M., Rosen, M., and Vickers, M. D. "An Open Comparison Between Routine and Self-Administered Postoperative Pain Relief." *Annals of the Royal College of Surgeons of England,* 1983, *65,* 18-19.

Sommer, R., and Ross, H. "Social Interaction on a Geriatric Ward." *International Journal of Social Psychiatry,* 1958, *4,* 128-133.

Sommer, R. *Tight Spaces.* Englewood Cliffs, N.J.: Prentice-Hall, 1974.

Spivak, M. "Sensory Distortions in Tunnels and Corridors." *Hospital and Community Psychiatry,* 1967, *18,* 24-30.

Stone, M. A., Stone, P. H., and Giffin, K. S. "Psychology of Office Design." *Texas Medicine,* 1990, *86*(1), 63-66.

Tagliacozzo, D. L. "The Nurse from the Patient's Point of View." In J. K. Skipper, Jr., and R. C. Leonard (eds.), *Social Interaction and Patient Care.* Philadelphia: Lippincott, 1965.

Tamsen, A., Hartvig, P., Fagerlund, C., and Dahlström, B. "Patient-Controlled Analgesic Therapy." *Clinical Pharmacy,* 1982, *7,* 149-175.

Tamsen, A., and others. "Patient Controlled Analgesic Therapy in the Early Postoperative Period." *Acta Anaesthesiology Scandinavia,* 1979, *23,* 462-470.

Taylor, A. G., Hudson, K., and Keeling, A. "Quality Nursing Care: The Consumers' Perspective Revisited." *Journal of Nursing Quality Assurance,* 1991, *5*(2), 23-31.

Teske, K., Daut, R. L., and Cleeland, C. S. "Relationships Between Nurses' Observations and Patients' Self-Reports About Pain." *Pain,* 1983, *16,* 289-296.

Thompson, J. D. "Patients Like These Four-Bed Wards." *Modern Hospitals,* 1955, *85*(6), 84-86.

Ulrich, R. S. "View Through a Window May Influence Recovery from Surgery." *Science,* 1984, *224,* 420-421.

Vaché, E. "Inadequate Treatment of Pain in Hospitalized Patients [letter]." *New England Journal of Medicine,* 1982, *307,* 55.

Weis, O. F., and others. "Attitudes of Patients, Housestaff, and Nurses Toward Postoperative Analgesic Care." *Anesthesia and Analgesia,* 1983, *62,* 70-74.

Winkel, G. H., and Holahan, C. J. "The Environmental Psychology of the Hospital: Is the Cure Worse than the Illness?" *Prevention in Human Services,* 1985-1986, *4,* 11-33.

7

Providing Effective
Emotional Support

Susan Edgman-Levitan

Sick people almost always want to get better. And getting better is accomplished in many ways—not the least of which is coping with the psychological, as well as the physical, demands of illness. "I will need more help with my mental recovery than with my physical problems," one patient told us. "Am I going to be an invalid?" she asked. "Will I ever dance again?" Most hospitalized patients feel vulnerable, isolated, and afraid. Many are forced, for the first time in their lives, to face their own mortality or the loss of a body part or function (Taylor, 1991). Lying in a hospital bed, many people find it hard to imagine coping with the normal activities of life at home or at work. Fears abound about the unknown course of illness and the permanent impairment it may cause. As Oliver Sacks put it in his book *Awakenings,* "The terrors of suffering, sickness and death, of losing ourselves and losing the world are the most elemental and intense we know; and so too are our dreams of recovery and rebirth, of being wonderfully restored to ourselves and the world" (1983, p. 202). Addressing the emotional component of illness is critical in a world where many conditions are chronic.

Hospitals and clinicians cannot afford to ignore patients' emotional needs. Increasingly, research demonstrates that patients' emotional states can influence the outcome of their illness. At Stanford University, Spiegel (1990) found that women with metastatic breast cancer who were enrolled in a support group lived twice as long as those in a control group matched for treatment protocols and severity of illness. A University of Minnesota study found that twelve out of thirteen severely depressed patients undergoing bone marrow transplant died within a year of the transplant, while 39 percent of the patients who were not depressed were still alive two years later (Goleman, 1991). Providing emotional support could prove to be more curative than some of the high-technology, expensive therapies currently employed.

Addressing patients' emotional needs can also be cost-effective. Patients who have such support leave the hospital earlier (Mumford, Schlesinger, and Glass, 1982; Devine and Cook, 1983), require less medication, begin walking again more quickly (Lawlis, Selby, Hinnant, and McCoy, 1985), are more satisfied with care, comply more readily with treatment regimens (Bohachick, 1984), and experience fewer side effects from drugs such as those administered during chemotherapy (Carey and Burish, 1987; Cotanch, 1987). Patients who learn relaxation techniques handle the stress of procedures or surgery better than other patients. Even brief training in progressive muscle relaxation techniques has alleviated nausea and vomiting in chemotherapy patients, decreased the need for pain medication in patients hospitalized for spinal surgery, and allowed the same patients to begin walking a full day earlier than patients treated in the typical postoperative fashion (Lawlis, Selby, Hinnant, and McCoy, 1985; Cobb, 1984; Bohachick, 1984).

Failure to address the psychological component of illness, whether acute or chronic, can also affect health status and the use of medical services. A patient's emotional response to illness may seriously affect the doctor-patient relationship and the treatments and medications prescribed. A patient's response to symptoms and to medical advice may also influence the subsequent management of illness and the patient's adherence to the prescribed regimen (Devine and Cook, 1983).

In this chapter, we shall present a taxonomy of social and emotional support and describe, from the patient's perspective, various approaches and methods hospitals can use to provide emotional support. These range from simple psychological support techniques designed to bolster self-esteem to sophisticated programs of support. While a comprehensive review of the research is beyond the scope of this chapter, we shall highlight important findings that help characterize the most effective methods.

Defining *Emotional Support*

"I remember very specifically when I was with the surgeon just prior to being operated on. He put his hand on my shoulder in such a way that it was extremely reassuring. That really was the best thing, and it sticks in my mind." The term *emotional support* evokes, for many of us, images of hand-holding, reassurance, or gentle solicitations of well-being. And for some patients, effective support may indeed be as simple as smiling or holding a hand, as it was for the focus-group patient quoted above. But addressing the fears and anxieties of many patients is more complicated than this, and health care professionals' efforts to be reassuring may even backfire. One cardiac patient, for example, described his doctors' efforts to "reassure" him about routine backup precautions for an invasive diagnostic imaging procedure: "[T]he surgeon comes over, and the doctor comes over, and say very nicely, 'You don't have to worry, we have a surgical team in the other room.' Well, wait a minute! If we have a surgical team in the other room, why *don't* I have to worry? I mean what are they [there] for? 'In case?' . . . Well, thanks, but. . . ."

Effective emotional support conveys a sense of genuine caring and concern for patients' needs, increases their ability to cope with their condition while they are in the hospital, contributes to their recovery or long-term management of their illness, and reassures them about the quality of care they are receiving. Some patients will need little more than a touch or a smile. Others may require intensive psychotherapy. Patients are very different in their needs, and their needs may change during the course of a hospitalization or an illness. Regardless, emotional support is an essential aspect of care for *all* patients, not just those who express a need for it or for whom nothing more can be done.

Emotional support, as we use the term here, overlaps with the concept of *social support* more commonly found in the literature. Several researchers have tried to give the concept more specificity. We believe that Wortman's taxonomy (1984) captures most of what patients tell us is important to them when they are in the hospital. Wortman defines support, emotional or social, as

- Expressing positive affect, including the sense that the sick person is cared for, loved, or esteemed
- Agreeing with, or acknowledging the appropriateness of, a patient's feelings, beliefs, or interpretations
- Encouraging the patient to express beliefs and feelings openly
- Providing advice or information or access to new and diverse information
- Providing tangible support, such as shopping, home care, or child care
- Giving the patient the sense of belonging to a network or support system of mutual obligation or reciprocal help

This taxonomy helps hospital staff, physicians, nurses, and families translate the general desire to be comforting and supportive into concrete, specific, and helpful actions. Encouraging family members to be physically present during critical discussions with the physician, for example, is more useful than simply admonishing them to be "supportive." Providing patients with realistic expectations about procedures is something doctors and nurses can do routinely that most patients will find helpful and reassuring. Statements like "I know how you are feeling" may be very comforting when they come from another patient but infuriating when made by a young healthy nurse. Hospitals that are clean, quiet, and well run convey a sense of safety and security that is reassuring to patients, even though such things do not usually come to mind when we think of providing emotional support.

We turn now to a discussion of the kinds of support patients consider helpful, bearing this taxonomy in mind.

What Patients Want

"That's really the feeling I got from the hospital, the day I walked in to when I left—that these were my friends. I was sick, and my friends were taking care of me." What specifically does it take to make patients feel that they are being cared for by friends as this patient did? Dakof and Taylor (1990) studied fifty-five cancer patients, in all stages of disease, to identify what, specifically, they found to be helpful or unhelpful, and from whom. Potential providers of support included spouses and other family members, friends, other cancer patients, nurses, and physicians. From the patients' perspective, the first and most important category of support was the expression of positive affect or bolstering of self-esteem. This included such actions as expressing concern and empathy, showing special understanding of the nature of the problem, calm acceptance of the problem, and the expression of optimism or hope. The majority of patients studied found expressions of love and encouragement to talk about feelings to be the *most* helpful support given by *all* providers; but it was *least* helpful when it was done poorly, or not at all. Forty percent of the patients queried complained that they received inadequate emotional support from physicians. As Rosenbaum observed in his preface to *The Doctor* (1988, p. vi), "When I became ill, like my patients, I wanted my doctors to be gods—and they couldn't be. But I also wanted them to understand my illness and my feelings and what I needed from my physicians. Those things they could have done—and some of them didn't."

Patients also attach considerable importance to the provision of *useful* information—the fourth item in Wortman's taxonomy, which we address more fully in earlier chapters on communication and information. This encompasses everything from giving patients specific information about upcoming tests and procedures to providing role models to help them cope with a chronic condition. It also includes giving patients realistic expectations about their illness, tests, and treatments. Patients in Dakof and Taylor's study also included optimism about prognosis and about their ability to live with the illness in the general category of "medical information." Thirty-eight percent of these patients thought that providing medical information was the most helpful thing physicians did for them, and 25 percent said that physicians were least helpful when they gave insufficient medical information. Twenty-seven percent found the expression of optimism as the most helpful physician behavior. Informing patients about mutual help, self-help, or appropriate support groups in the community may also be invaluable for their long-term adjustment to health problems.

How Patients' Needs Differ

As the following quotations illustrate, patients differ both in the type of support they need and in the methods they find most useful: "They had no idea what this patient, in this bed—scared to death—was thinking, with all these things you're hearing around you, and the equipment. . . . They're talking to each other like you're not even there." "I'm one of those people who, if I'm faced with a situation like surgery, I accept it, and I feel that it's out of my hands, almost."

Clinicians are adept at characterizing patients' physiological processes when they plan diagnostic and treatment protocols. The same care should be taken in determining how to offer emotional support and when it is helpful. Patients vary in their coping styles and in their perceptions of control over what happens to them. And these differences have important implications for the kind of emotional support that is most helpful.

Styles of Coping with Stress

Researchers in the field describe what they call *problem-focused* and *emotion-focused* styles of coping with stress. Problem-focused behaviors entail confronting the problem, seeking information about how to manage it, and devising strategies to deal with it. Emotion-focused strategies often entail denial and escape or avoidance, or reconfiguring the problem to make it more positive. Most people use both strategies to deal with stress, but one style usually predominates. Several studies have shown that patients who use problem-focused techniques make better adjustments and have better outcomes than those who use avoidance and denial (Dakof and Taylor, 1990; Solomon, 1991; Temoshok and others, 1985; Kneier and Temoshok, 1984; Temoshok, 1985; Scheier, Weintraub, and Carver, 1986; Carver and Gaines, 1987; Scheier and Carver, 1987). In fact, the positive effects of optimism on outcome and adjustment are attributed, in part, to optimists' use of problem-focused strategies.

Temoshok has also documented the negative effects of emotion-focused styles among melanoma patients at the cellular level of immune function (Kneier and Temoshok, 1984; Temoshok, 1985).

Other researchers have characterized individuals as "sensitizers," "avoiders" or "repressors," or "neutrals" in their styles of coping and processing information (Williams and Kendall, 1985). So-called "sensitizers" admit to negative emotions, "avoiders" or "repressors" deny them, and "neutrals" admit to both behaviors. Studies of patients undergoing surgery, endoscopy, and other painful or unpleasant procedures at Veterans' Administration hospitals (Andrew, 1970; Shipley, Butt, and Horwitz, 1979; Shipley, Butt, Horwitz, and Farbry, 1978; Leventhal and Everhart, 1979) have demonstrated that "sensitizers" or "neutrals" recover more quickly and have less anxiety when they are given as much information as possible about what to expect. On the other hand, "avoiders" who are given such extensive information actually have more anxiety, require more medication, and have worse outcomes.

Patients also vary a great deal in their perception of how much control they have over their lives. People with a strong internal "locus of control" feel the need to exert influence over what happens to them. They believe they are responsible for what happens to them through their own efforts to control the situation. Those with an external "locus of control" tend, on the other hand, to hold outside institutions, other people, or "fate" responsible for what happens to them. Several studies have shown that people who perceive control as external to themselves resemble "avoiders" in their need for information, while those with a strong internal locus of control do better with detailed information about what to expect. In a study of patients undergoing oral surgery, Auerbach, Kendall, Cuttler, and Levitt (1976) found that subjects with internal control who were given specific information prior to surgery adjusted better than those with external control who received the same information. Subjects with external control adjusted better when they received, instead, general information about the facility.

Assessing Patients and Targeting Their Needs

Assessing patients' coping styles or their perceptions of control requires neither a great deal of time nor special training. Patients are forthcoming about what kind of preparation they need, if asked. As one focus-group patient candidly admitted, "People need different kinds of information. Some need it all. I'm not sure I need it all. . . . Sometimes you're better off not knowing too much." Self-reporting instruments that can be used to assess locus of control, preferred coping styles, and level of anxiety already exist. Elective patients could be evaluated using such instruments as part of the preadmission process, and emergency admissions could be assessed by the nursing staff, as appropriate. It is also helpful simply to talk with patients to find out what kind of emotional support they find helpful, how much they know about their illness or about any procedure or surgery they might face, and how anxious and fearful they are. Friends and family members, too, are often quite knowledgeable about patients' coping styles and preferences. Such structured discussions would also create opportunities to introduce patients and their families to chaplaincy services and other available sources of support.

In addition, hospitals might consider developing different kinds of educational materials for different kinds of patients. While "sensitizers" and "neutrals" might be given detailed information about the risks and benefits of upcoming procedures to help them prepare for the experience, "avoiders" should probably be spared the excruciating details and might be given, instead, information that minimizes the danger and maximizes trust in the competence of the providers. Differences in patients' emotional coping styles must also be taken into account when informing them about living wills and advance directives, as required by the Patient Self-Determination Act. Although the purpose of the act is to give patients more say about what happens to them, both the timing and the manner of its implementation may be unnecessarily upsetting.

Timing

Patients' needs for support also vary depending on where they are in the course of an illness. Newly diagnosed cancer patients, for example, may have multiple needs: reassurance from health care providers, love and affection from family members, information about treatment options from physicians, and practical information from other cancer patients about what to expect. Terminal patients, on the other hand, usually have specific needs for tangible support with pain control and activities of daily living. Patients awaiting an elective surgical procedure may need reassurance about the experience of anesthesia, along with relaxation techniques to help control preoperative anxiety. After surgery, their needs will be quite different. Patients with chronic illness will have different emotional needs during a remission than in the midst of a full-scale flare-up of the disease.

Providing Emotional Support in the Hospital

In the hospital, many factors influence a patient's emotional state and providers should consider a variety of approaches to reduce stress and relieve anxiety.

The Hospital Environment

According to Greenfield, "They [hospitals] and their technological equipment operate against a background of remorseless human shortcoming, bureaucratic inefficiency and indifference. That, not some need to understand the exotic equipment or science, is the problem. What is required is a fundamental, painstaking re-education process on the part of the whole institution—a relearning of attentiveness, individual accountability, care" (1986, p. 74).

From the patient's perspective, hospitals are often cold, intimidating places. They smell strange, the lights are always on, and equipment—menacing and certainly foreign—litters the hallway and the patient's room. Sounds are frightening and unusual, and helplessness leaves one constantly alert to any changes outside the door that may announce the arrival of bad news, more pain, or both. Patients respond emotionally to the people who care for them and to their environment. Hospital managers may not be able to control the behavior of physicians, family members, or other visitors, but they can set the tone through the values they model and reward in the staff who do report to them and through the physical ambience they try to create.

Sick, worried patients are especially vulnerable to first impressions. The security guards who greet them in the parking areas and at the entrances may be gracious and helpful, or they may be bullying. One maternity patient related the following story: "I arrived at the hospital in labor with my first child. We frantically parked our car in the emergency room parking lot. As we jumped out, the security guard came up to us and—much to our surprise—wished us well and went to get me a wheelchair. We thought he was going to scold us for disobeying some hospital rule. I took it as a good omen and knew I was in good hands and everything would be all right." Patients are reassured by well-attended, clean public spaces and by reception areas and admitting offices staffed by knowledgeable, courteous people who enjoy working with the public.

Everyone who comes in contact with hospital patients has the potential to influence them emotionally, for good or for ill. As one focus-group patient told us, "The housekeeper . . . has the same ability to come in and warm up the room with friendliness as the surgeon does. In my case, a very nice guy came two days in a row, and we joked a little bit. I had a lot better experience from him than I did with the intern poking me." Clinical staff may become inured to clutter and noise that, to patients, connote disorder, confusion, unknown tortures. "In the same building with the state-of-the-art machine that can see your brain and hear your blood are the crumpled Kleenexes and old dressings that should have been disposed of, all lying there under the unconcerned eye of the technical assistant who is thinking mainly of lunch" (Greenfield, 1986, p. 74). Guest excellence programs that are tailored to all levels of the hospital's work force may help convey this point to all staff. But care must also be taken at all levels of staff recruitment to hire competent and friendly people suited for work in an environment with sick people.

Crisis Intervention

People who become seriously ill are often thrown into a state of emotional crisis. One patient described her own reaction to a diagnosis of breast cancer: "When the doctor called to tell me, I was overwhelmed with terror. I didn't think I would ever sleep again.

Driving to the doctor's office the next day, I watched people getting
on buses, walking down the sidewalk chatting, and felt as if a plate-
glass wall had fallen between me and the rest of the world. My side
was silent—like death—without laughter or life. I was terrified and
incapable of looking beyond the next moment. I wanted to jump
out of my life into a fantasy world." Auerbach and Kilmann (1977)
distinguished between "ordinarily functioning individuals who [re-
spond] with disabling levels of anxiety to discrete environmental
stressors" and "chronically maladjusted individuals whose behavior
. . . stems from a continuing psychiatric disorder." For the former
group, crisis intervention techniques may be a useful form of emotional support. "Crisis therapy focuses on resolution of immediate
problems and emotional conflicts, as opposed to restructuring of
basic personality" (p. 1190).

One intervention using crisis therapy techniques for cancer patients might well be adapted for any patient in crisis (Rickel, 1987).
The intervention aims to take problems that seem to be "mountains"
from the patient's perspective and to make them manageable. At the
first step of the intervention, health care providers gather information
from the patient or family about several dimensions of daily living:
physical, intellectual, emotional, social, and material. The next step
is to pose two concrete questions to the patient or family: "What was
the last straw?" and "What do you want me [the provider] to do?" The
patient and provider then separately list the problems each thinks is
paramount. The patient groups the problems into three categories:
(1) "things I can change soon," (2) "things I may be able to change
in time," and (3) "things I cannot change." The health care provider
also groups the problems into three categories: (1) problems that are
life threatening, (2) problems the provider can fix, and (3) problems
that should be referred to someone else. Following this exercise, the
patient and provider "build a mountain" with the problem list, putting the most manageable ones on top. Although this exercise is
suggested for nurses and patients, it might also be used by physicians,
social workers, or therapists.

Information Giving

Most patients know very little about the actual experience of illness,
technical procedures, or surgery. Giving them information about
the sensory aspect of such experiences helps reduce their anxiety and

distress. Johnson and colleagues (Johnson and Leventhal, 1974; Johnson, Rice, Fuller, and Endress, 1978; Johnson, Christman, and Stitt, 1985) have conducted studies to examine the effect of different types of information on the reduction of distress in patients undergoing various invasive medical procedures, such as endoscopy. She concludes that inaccurate expectations about the physical sensations of such procedures are the critical source of distress for most patients. Patients will be less fearful undergoing a procedure, she suggests, if they have a clear understanding of how it will feel.

The standard written or audiotaped preparatory instructions patients are given prior to undergoing technical procedures might therefore incorporate a description of sensations one might expect. However, such descriptions should avoid subjective descriptions of how distressing or upsetting the sensations might be, since this will be different for each patient. In one study, children waiting for cast removal were given several different types of information about what to expect. One group was given an audiotape that included the sound of the saw and a description of the heat and flying plaster dust. Another group was given a narrative description of the removal process. And a third group was given no information at all. The children who were given sensory as well as factual information about the process exhibited the least distress about the procedure (Leventhal and Everhart, 1979).

In their quantitative review of the effects of psychological interventions on recovery from surgery and heart attacks, Mumford, Schlesinger, and Glass (1982) found that educational approaches that combined factual information about patients' clinical condition with short-term psychological interventions designed to provide reassurance, reduce "irrational" beliefs, and relieve anxiety had a positive impact on patients' speed of recovery, posthospital complications, and cooperation with medical treatment in the hospital. Most of these interventions were modest in scope and were apparently effective even though they were not matched to the patients' coping styles.

Relaxation and Stress Reduction

Many hospitals have experimented with the use of progressive muscle relaxation therapy to help patients cope with the stress of cardiac rehabilitation (Bohachick, 1984), back surgery (Lawlis, Selby, Hinnant, and McCoy, 1985), side effects of chemotherapy (Cotanch, 1987; Carey and Burish, 1987; Cobb, 1984), and the general stress of hospitalization. Progressive muscle relaxation therapy is easy to teach and relatively easy to learn. Some programs augment sessions conducted by a professional therapist with the use of audiotapes, others use audiotapes only, and still others use a combination of trained volunteers and audiotapes. Programs that combined professional instruction with audiotapes have been found most effective in reducing anxiety and side effects, perhaps because volunteers are more likely to be distracted by the chaos and turmoil in the hospital environment (Carey and Burish, 1987). In their studies of the use of progressive muscle relaxation therapy to reduce the side effects of chemotherapy, Carey and Burish (1987) and Cotanch (1987) found that proper training by a professional was necessary to attain the desired results. Once patients have been trained, most request audiotapes as an aid to relaxation, to help them focus on the technique and block out environmental distractions.

Lawlis, Selby, Hinnant, and McCoy (1985), investigating the effects of relaxation instruction on preoperative spinal surgery patients, found that the relaxation group had a length of stay two days shorter and requested one-third the amount of pain medication when compared with a control group receiving no such instruction. The experimental relaxation group was given a three-hour course prior to admission that covered the nature of pain and the role of endorphins in pain relief, deep breathing and distraction techniques, and training in progressive muscle relaxation. Patients were also offered individual instruction following the course, but none requested it.

Careful attention to roommate assignment can also be used to reduce preoperative anxiety and provide reassurance. Kulik and Mahler (1987) found that preoperative cardiac surgery patients assigned to rooms with postoperative general or cardiac surgery patients had less anxiety prior to surgery, ambulated twice as much, and left the hospital 1.4 days earlier than a control group. The researchers postulated that postoperative patients and their families are less anxious than preoperative patients, thereby reducing the "contagion effect" of anxiety, and that postoperative patients provide living proof that one can survive serious surgery. Kulik and

Mahler also noted that experienced patients provide salient information about the sensations associated with surgery and specific suggestions about how to cope with postoperative problems.

Implementing such a matched roommate program may be difficult in a busy hospital where available beds are few. Moreover, many patients are now admitted the morning of their surgery. However, there may be ways to apply the lessons of this program by using experienced patients as resources. The "Patient-to-Patient, Heart-to-Heart" Program at Boston's Beth Israel Hospital is one such model. In this case, cancer patients who have undergone treatment are paired with newly diagnosed patients or with those who are about to undergo a new therapy or procedure. The experienced patients, all of whom have been trained by an experienced oncology social worker, provide the others with whatever information they request. Visits can take place prior to admission, in the hospital, or after the patient goes home. The interaction may consist of a phone call, one visit, or an ongoing relationship, at the discretion of the patient and volunteer. The University of Utah Hospital also uses former patients as the principal "stars" of videotapes sent home with recovering patients. In addition, preoperative information sessions conducted by patients and professionals might provide patients and their families with a wealth of information about what to expect in the hospital and after discharge.

Emotional Support Outside the Hospital: Support and Self-Help Groups

"I needed to find someone immediately who knew my terror; someone I could talk with on a personal—rather than clinical—level; someone who had 'been there.' I needed to find a survivor." This quotation from Mullan and Hoffman's almanac of resources for cancer survivors (1990, p. 86), shows that patients need emotional support not only while they are in the hospital but also after they leave, when they face the long-term task of adjustment, treatment, or recovery. Groups composed of patients with similar diagnoses are widely used to help provide this ongoing support. Although they differ widely in composition, structure, and philosophy, all of the groups broadly designated as *support groups* exist to provide help or address problems that are not routinely addressed by medical professionals. Dean (1986) distinguishes three categories of such groups: (1) those that operate within the health care system, based on professional therapeutic concepts; (2) those that operate in cooperation with, or parallel to, the health care system, using group members or health care professionals to provide services that are not regularly available within the system; and (3) those that operate in opposition to the conventional health care system, rejecting standard medical theories, practices, and approaches to care. Generally speaking, the term *support group* is used to apply to professionally run groups that fall into the first or second of Dean's categories, while *self-help groups* are, by definition, not run by professionals and fall into the second or third category.

Support Groups: Professionals and Patients Working Together

Professionally run support groups for patients, or for families of patients, with such chronic illnesses as cancer and cardiac disease are fairly common. Similar groups for the families of patients with chronic neurological disease such as Alzheimer's are also often established. They provide a haven for group members to discuss their problems coping with or managing their illness. In other respects, however, support groups are not all the same. Some may be informal drop-in sessions run by nursing staff, meeting at a set time and place on an inpatient unit (Hyler, Corley, and McMahon, 1985; Lombardo, Cave, and Naso, 1988; Kopel and Mock, 1978; Sellshopp, Ludeke, and Haertel, 1981). Inpatient groups tend to have a revolving membership, because of the brief lengths of stay of most patients, and they therefore serve mostly for brief psychological support and information giving. Such groups can help identify patients or family members who might benefit from individual counseling or group support in an outpatient setting. They also serve to identify areas of misunderstanding between staff and patients and improve communication. For example, some family members or patients have serious misunderstandings about treatment options or the interpretation of test results that can be corrected, once they are identified. Sometimes staff receive important information about problems on a unit or in the hospital that they might otherwise miss without an organized forum in which patients can express their concerns or ask for help.

Other types of support groups may be regularly scheduled outpatient groups that resemble group therapy sessions, while still others will combine a structured curriculum teaching useful skills with psychological support from other patients and a trained facilitator (Kabat-Zinn, 1991; Cunningham and others, 1991).

Many hospitals, as well as advocacy organizations like the American Cancer Society, the Arthritis Foundation, and the American Heart Association, offer regularly scheduled outpatient support groups for a number of different health problems. These groups, led by a professional facilitator such as a nurse, social worker, or psychologist, offer concrete information about the illness, emotional support, and practical information about coping with the particular medical problem in daily living. A smaller number of support groups are designed around a formal curriculum that teaches patients different techniques for coping with chronic illness. To help with depression and fear, these groups usually emphasize training in relaxation or meditation techniques, guided imagery or visualization, and psychological techniques such as cognitive restructuring. Time is also made available for members to share information, thoughts, and feelings. Groups that emphasize these formal skills are usually led by trained physicians or psychologists, perhaps with the assistance of patients who can serve as role models and provide practical information.

The Stress Reduction and Relaxation Program at the University of Massachusetts Medical Center in Worcester has trained over 4,000 people in an eight-week program described as "an intensive self-directed training program in the art of conscious living," drawing on a form of meditation originally developed within the Buddhist traditions of Asia. Kabat-Zinn borrows a line from the movie *Zorba the Greek* to describe realities of living that bring patients to the stress reduction program. Asked if he has ever been married, Zorba replies, "Am I not a man? Of course I've been married! Wife, house, kids, everything! *The full catastrophe!*" (Kabat-Zinn, 1991, p. 7). The Stress Reduction Program aims to help people embrace the "full catastrophe" by helping them see themselves and the world differently, work with their bodies, thoughts, feelings, and perceptions in a new way, and laugh at themselves and the world around them (Kabat-Zinn, 1991; Moyers, 1993).

The Section on Behavioral Medicine at the Deaconess Hospital in Boston offers support groups for patients with cancer, AIDS, fertility problems, and other chronic conditions. The groups are co-led by a psychologist and a physician and last for eight weeks each. Training in the relaxation response is provided, along with practical information about other stress reduction techniques, nutrition, yoga, cognitive restructuring, and living with a chronic illness. Commonweal, a health service and research institute in Bolinas, California, offers an innovative week-long health promotion program for cancer patients and their families that combines emotional support techniques with intensive training in meditation, yoga, nutrition and other complementary cancer therapies, and other information for cancer survivors (Lerner and Remen, 1987; Moyers, 1993).

Support groups led by professionally trained staff are generally more respected by referring medical professionals, who are reassured that the course content will be appropriate to the needs of the patients. Trained professionals are also more likely to provide reliable, up-to-date information, to correct mistaken assumptions, to competently handle the difficult emotional issues that may arise, and to recognize patients who require more intensive individual therapy or medical intervention. Most of these groups also provide training in coping skills that benefit group members, above and beyond the emotional support they gain. The hospital affiliation of many professionally run support groups further enhances their esteem among medical professionals.

However, professionally led support groups are not without their drawbacks. Trained hired professionals are expensive, and group fees can be quite high, ranging from about $500 per course to over a $1,000 for some short-term residential programs. While some insurance plans cover the costs of support groups, many do not. Most groups also meet during the day, when working people, parents of small children, and others caring for dependent family members find it difficult to attend. Moreover, groups tend only to be available for patients or the relatives of patients with life-threatening or severely disabling diseases. Many programs also fail to take into account cultural differences in response to pain or serious illness. They often cater to a middle-class, well-educated clientele, with a high degree of openness to stress reduction techniques that others see as somewhat offbeat, a familiarity with the language and methods of therapy, and comfort with emotional expression. Moreover, time limitations may not allow adequate opportunity to deal with emotional issues evoked during the meetings, and the typical six- to eight-week time frame may be too brief for some patients to learn the skills. Nor do hospitals routinely collect information about support groups available to patients. Sometimes just finding a group requires a tremendous amount of tenacity and resourcefulness on the part of a patient or a family member already struggling to cope with illness.

Self-Help Groups

Self-help groups, by definition, are composed only of people sharing a common problem. They do not rely on professionals for leadership or training (Stewart, 1990; Robinson, 1978; Dean, 1986). Although health care professionals may look askance at these lay groups or at best view their services as marginal in importance, patients often seek them out on their own and, in fact, use professional health care as supplemental (Dean, 1986). As one member of a self-help group for patients with serious dermatological disease explained, "It's important to have a place where you don't have to hide, where you can be yourself" (Lombardo, Cave, and Naso, 1988). Participants in self-help groups often report that the groups help "boost psychological morale, self-esteem, and coping abilities" (Cousins, 1989, p. 241). As Cousins explains, "Just as the brain tends to convert bad news into panic and helplessness, so strong support from family and friends can help maintain or restore emotional equilibrium" (p. 280). Hospitals, physicians, and other health care providers need to develop a better understanding of the needs these groups address and either develop their own support groups or establish strong referral sources for groups run within the community.

Hospitals can learn about self-help groups by contacting self-help clearinghouses around the country and by talking with organizations that advocate for different types of patients, such as the Arthritis Foundation and the American Heart Association.

Summary

Illness imposes an emotional and psychological burden on patients and their families that is often as heavy as the physical one. When these needs are acknowledged and addressed, patients suffer less and get better faster. What they need are genuine expressions of concern and caring—from those they love and from the doctors, nurses, and others caring for them. They also need the chance to express their own beliefs, feelings, and fears, however extreme or "irrational" they may seem; information that is accurate, appropriate, and useful; and a sense that they are a continuing and vital part of a social community. Developing appropriate strategies to address these needs requires sensitivity to the variations in individual styles of coping with stress, to the patient's underlying emotional state, and to changing needs over the course of an illness. Most people understand what they want, need, and can handle, but the emotional crisis of illness can seriously compromise their usual resiliency. Strategies that hospitals and other providers can use to help address the emotional and psychological components of illness include eliminating or softening the stressors in the hospital environment, training staff in techniques of crisis intervention, and developing informational materials appropriate to patients' varying needs and styles of coping. Other desirable strategies include offering programs of relaxation and stress reduction to identified groups of patients and providing patients with ongoing support outside the hospital through referrals to support groups and self-help groups.

Suggestions for Improvement

- Use simple progressive muscle relaxation techniques to help patients cope with medication side effects or difficult procedures. Use closed-circuit television to provide information about such techniques and their use.

- Offer patients an audiotape player with earphones, along with a variety of musical, comedy, or relaxation tapes.
- Encourage doctors and nurses to review with patients the kind of information, assistance, and support they need and the approaches they find most helpful. Make this a routine part of the history and physical or the nursing assessment.
- Develop educational materials suited to patients' varied coping styles.
- Use focus groups or other methods of eliciting feedback from different types of patients to develop appropriate protocols and materials for administering the Patient Self-Determination Act.
- Plan services and programs with the same concern for patients' psychological and emotional needs that is devoted to their physical requirements. Use focus groups and other methods of patient involvement to plan programs and services appropriate to specific diagnostic groups.
- Give all patients general information on chaplaincy services.
- Develop a network of patients and family members willing to share their experiences with newly diagnosed patients and their families.
- Give patients written information about support groups and self-help clearinghouses. The *Self-Help Sourcebook* may be purchased from the American Self-Help Clearinghouse, St. Clares-Riverside Medical Center, Denville, New Jersey 07834, (201) 625-7101.

References

Andrew, J. M. "Recovery from Surgery With and Without Preparatory Instruction, for Three Coping Styles." *Journal of Personality and Social Psychology,* 1970, *15,* 223–226.

Auerbach, S. M., Kendall, P. C., Cuttler, H. F., and Levitt, N. R. "Anxiety, Locus of Control, Type of Preparatory Information, and Adjustment to Dental Surgery." *Journal of Consulting and Clinical Psychology,* 1976, *44,* 809–818.

Auerbach, S. M., and Kilmann, P. R. "Crisis Intervention: A Review of Outcome Research." *Psychological Bulletin,* 1977, *84,* 1189–1217.

Bohachick, P. "Progressive Relaxation Training in Cardiac Rehabilitation: Effect on Psychologic Variables." *Nursing Research,* 1984, *33,* 283–287.

Carey, M. P., and Burish, T. G. "Providing Relaxation Training to Cancer Chemotherapy Patients: A Comparison of Three Delivery Techniques." *Journal of Consulting and Clinical Psychology,* 1987, *55,* 732–737.

Carver, C. S., and Gaines, J. G. "Optimism, Pessimism, and Postpartum Depression." *Cognitive Therapy and Research,* 1987, *4,* 449–462.

Cobb, S. C. "Teaching Relaxation Techniques to Cancer Patients." *Cancer Nursing,* 1984, *7,* 157–161.

Cotanch, P. "Progressive Muscle Relaxation as Antiemetic Therapy for Cancer Patients." *Oncology Nursing Forum,* 1987, *14,* 33–37.

Cousins, N. *Head First: The Biology of Hope.* New York: Dutton, 1989.

Cunningham, A., and others. "A Group Psychoeducational Program to Help Cancer Patients Cope with and Combat Their Disease." *Advances: The Journal of Mind-Body Health,* 1991, *7,* 41–56.

Dakof, G. A., and Taylor, S. E. "Victims' Perceptions of Social Support: What Is Helpful from Whom?" *Journal of Personality and Social Psychology,* 1990, *58,* 80–89.

Dean, K. "Lay Care in Illness." *Social Science in Medicine,* 1986, *22,* 275–284.

Devine, E. C., and Cook, T. D. "A Meta-Analytic Analysis of Effects of Psychoeducational Interventions on Length of Postsurgical Hospital Stay." *Nursing Research,* 1983, *32,* 267–274.

Goleman, D. "Doctors Find Comfort Is a Potent Medicine." *New York Times,* November 26, 1991, p. C1.

Greenfield, M. "The Land of Hospital." *Newsweek,* June 30, 1986, p. 74.

Hyler, B. J., Corley, M. C., and McMahon, D. "The Role of Nursing in a Support Group for Heart Transplantation Recipients and Their Families." *The Journal of Heart Transplantation,* 1985, *4,* 453–456.

Johnson, J., Christman, N. J., and Stitt, C. "Personal Control Interventions: Short- and Long-Term Effects on Surgical Patients." *Research in Nursing and Health,* 1985, *8,* 131–145.

Johnson, J., and Leventhal, H. "Effects of Accurate Expectations and Behavioral Instructions on Reactions During a Noxious Medical Examination." *Journal of Personality and Social Psychology,* 1974, *29,* 710–718.

Johnson, J. J., Rice, V. H., Fuller, S. S., and Endress, M. P. "Sensory Information, Instruction in a Coping Strategy, and Recovery from Surgery." *Research in Nursing and Health,* 1978, *1,* 4–17.

Kabat-Zinn, J. *Full Catastrophe Living.* New York: Dell, 1991.

Kneier, A. W., and Temoshok, L. "Regressive Coping Reactions in Patients with Malignant Melanoma as Compared to Cardiovascular Disease Patients." *Journal of Psychosomatic Research,* 1984, *28,* 145–155.

Kopel, K., and Mock, L. A. "The Use of Group Sessions for the Emotional Support of Families of Terminal Patients." *Death Education,* 1978, *1,* 409–422.

Kulik, J. A., and Mahler, H.I.M. "Effects of Preoperative Roommate Assignment on Preoperative Anxiety and Recovery from Coronary-Bypass Surgery." *Health Psychology,* 1987, *6,* 525–543.

Lawlis, G. F., Selby, D., Hinnant, D., and McCoy, C. E. "Reduction of Postoperative Pain Parameters by Presurgical Relaxation Instructions for Spinal Pain Patients." *Spine,* 1985, *10,* 649–651.

Lerner, M., and Remen, R. N. "Tradecraft of the Commonweal Cancer Help Program." *Advances: The Journal of Mind-Body Health,* 1987, *4,* 11–25.

Leventhal, H., and Everhart, D. "Emotion, Pain, and Physical Illness." In C. E. Izard (ed.), *Emotions in Personality and Psychopathology.* New York: Plenum, 1979.

Lombardo, B. A., Cave, L. A., and Naso, S. "Use of a Support Group for Dermatologic Patients." *Cutis,* 1988, *41,* 121–123.

Moyers, B. D. *Healing and the Mind.* New York: Doubleday, 1993.

Mullan, F., and Hoffman, B., *An Almanac of Practical Resources for Cancer Survivors.* Mt. Vernon, New York: Consumer Reports Books, 1990.

Mumford, E., Schlesinger, H. J., and Glass, G. V. "The Effects of Psychological Intervention on Recovery from Surgery and Heart

Attacks: An Analysis of the Literature." *American Journal of Public Health*, 1982, *72*, 141–151.

Rickel, L. "Making Mountains Manageable: Maximizing Quality of Life Through Crisis Intervention." *Oncology Nursing Forum*, 1987, *14*, 29–34.

Robinson, D. "Self-Help Groups." *British Journal of Hospital Medicine*, 1978, *20*, 306–311.

Rosenbaum, E. E. *The Doctor*. New York: Ballantine Books, 1988.

Sacks, O. *Awakenings*. New York: Dutton, 1983.

Scheier, M. F., and Carver, C. S. "Dispositional Optimism and Physical Well Being: The Influence of Generalized Outcome Expectancies on Health." *Journal of Personality*, 1987, *55*, 169–210.

Scheier, M. F., Weintraub, J. K., and Carver, C. S. "Coping with Stress: Divergent Strategies of Optimists and Pessimists." *Journal of Personality and Social Psychology*, 1986, *51*, 1257–1264.

Sellshopp, A., Ludeke, H., and Haertel, G. "Structure and Functions of the Heidelberg University Organisation for After-Care of Cancer Patients." *Psychotherapy and Psychosomatics*, 1981, *36*, 17–23.

Shipley, R. H., Butt, J. H., Horwitz, B., and Farbry, J. E. "Preparation for a Stressful Medical Procedure: Effect of Amount of Stimulus Preexposure and Coping Style." *Journal of Consulting and Clinical Psychology*, 1978, *46*, 499–507.

Shipley, R. H., Butt, J. H., and Horwitz, E. A. "Preparation to Reexperience a Stressful Medical Examination: Effect of Repetitious Videotape Exposure and Coping Style." *Journal of Consulting and Clinical Psychology*, 1979, *47*, 485–492.

Solomon, G. F., Temoshok, L., O'Leary, A., and Zich, J. "An Intensive Psychoimmunologic Study of Long-Surviving Persons with AIDS." *Annals of the New York Academy of Science*, 1987, *496*, 647–655.

Spiegel, D. "Can Psychotherapy Prolong Cancer Survival?" *Psychosomatics*, 1990, *31*, 361–365.

Stewart, M. J. "Expanding Theoretical Conceptualizations of Self-Help Groups." *Social Science in Medicine*, 1990, *31*, 1057–1066.

Taylor, S. "Hospital Patient Behavior: Reactance, Helplessness, or Control." In H. S. Friedman and R. M. DiMatteo (eds.), *Inter-*

personal Issues in Health Care. San Diego, Calif.: Academic Press, 1991.

Temoshok, L. "Biopsychosocial Studies on Cutaneous Malignant Melanoma: Psychosocial Factors Associated with Prognostic Indicators, Progression, Psychophysiology, and Tumor-Host Response." *Social Science in Medicine,* 1985, *20,* 833–840.

Temoshok, L., and others. "The Relationship of Psychosocial Factors to Prognostic Indicators in Cutaneous Malignant Melanoma." *Journal of Psychosomatic Research,* 1985, *29,* 139–153.

Williams, C. L., and Kendall, P. C. "Psychological Aspects of Patient Education for Stressful Medical Procedures." *Health Education Quarterly,* 1985, *12,* 135–150.

Wortman, C. B. "Social Support and the Cancer Patient." *Cancer,* 1984, *53* (Supplement), 2339–2362.

8

Involving and Supporting Family and Friends

Beth Ellers

Family members, close friends, and "significant others" can have a far greater impact on patients' experience of illness, and on their long-term health and happiness, than any health care professional. Friends and relatives take care of the patients, especially when they are home. They offer love and encouragement. They may cook meals, look after children, handle the shopping, pay bills, or take on any of the myriad responsibilities of daily life that a sick person cannot fulfill. They often convince the patients to seek medical help and then steer them through the receptionists, triage nurses, doctors, billing and insurance offices, and other hurdles of the health care system. They are the eyes and ears that watch over patients and report what they see to doctors and nurses. They remind patients to take medications and follow treatment regimens. And through their own behavior, they profoundly influence the lifetime habits that affect the patients' well-being over the longer run. Edward Rosenbaum, in his book, *The Doctor,* described how his own experience of illness made him long for and appreciate his mother's care, years after she had died. "At seventy years of age I still wanted my mother at my side to nurse me. . . . Once she undertook a patient's care, she never left that person's side. . . . She monitored the doctor's orders, the diets, the nursing care, and the patient. Many doctors and nurses are disturbed by such meddlesome family members, and at times I felt embarrassed by my mother's interference. I thought she was overreacting and being too motherly. But today I know that she was right" (1988, p. 31).

Although health care providers may be accustomed to thinking of family in terms of "next of kin," the concept must be expanded these days to include anyone the *patient* recognizes to be a significant relative, friend, or companion with a legitimate and genuine interest in that person's well-being and care, regardless of biological or legal relationships. Throughout this chapter, we use the term *family* in its broadest sense to include those significant relationships.

Family involvement is critical to patient-centered care. Yet serious illness throws a monkey wrench into any family that makes it hard even to carry on as usual, much less provide the extraordinary help and support a sick person requires. And health care institutions in this country often create barriers between patients and their families that make it even more difficult for families to offer their support—a practice that would be regarded as "very strange behavior indeed" in other parts of the world (Darbyshire, 1987, p. 23).

In this chapter, we explore the functions families serve and the realities they face in their role as caregivers or care partners, as long-term promoters of health and well-being, and as providers of essential social and emotional support (Fleming, 1987). We examine these dimensions of family involvement from the point of view of the patient, the family, and the provider or health care institution—distinct though overlapping and sometimes conflicting perspectives. And finally, we review programs and interventions that help health care providers and institutions accommodate families in their dual role as users and providers of health services. These range from radical restructuring of health services to relatively simple, inexpensive activities that address specific needs.

Why Involve Families?

Families play many different roles during a patient's illness.

Patients depend on their families to look out for their interests. One of the most important functions of family members from the patient's perspective, according to the patients in our focus groups, is to serve as proxy decision makers and as advocates to negotiate the administrative system and cut through bureaucratic red tape. Because the patients are often too incapacitated to look out for themselves, they rely heavily on friends and family members to look out for them. "'Be a pain in the neck,' the nurse advised, knowing from experience what works. . . . Being a pain in the neck is nature's way of getting answers" (DeLeon, 1991, p. 2B).

Serving as patient advocate may at times put family members in an adversarial role with health care providers. When families feel frustrated with the care or with the system, they may indeed respond by being "a pain in the neck." Health care providers may regard these families as a nuisance, although they may be performing an important service for the patient. In one study of family interactions with providers in emergency rooms, nearly one-half of the nurses viewed families as "potentially troublesome, . . . demanding, meddlesome, [and] overreactive" (Darbyshire, 1987, p. 24). Health care providers often act on such perceptions by restricting family access, limiting visitation hours, or withholding information, justifying these actions on the grounds that visitors interfere with staff routines and disturb the patient's rest (Darbyshire, 1987).

Patients need families to be involved in care and decision making. "I have found from familial experience in hospitals that you have to follow . . . your mother or father or son or whatever . . . —how they are supposed to be medicated, what they're supposed to get at night—because I think it's very dangerous to leave it to the nurses." As this remark from a family member of a focus-group patient suggests, one of the responsibilities family members feel most acutely is the obligation to monitor the patient's care and to participate in decisions about their care. And what family members complain about most is the lack of information (Mayou, Foster, and Williamson, 1978; Northouse, 1988), support (Lewis, 1986), and recognition for their role. Families want to be kept informed about the patient's condition, progress, and prognosis and to be consulted when there are important decisions to be made. As one family member remarked, "We were beginning to feel more like accessories than participants in the medical process" (DeLeon, 1991, p. 2B).

As part of our national survey of hospitalized patients, we

asked over 2,000 individuals identified as the patients' "care partners" if the providers had adequately involved them in decisions about the patients' care. While 75 percent of the care partners responded that they were involved the right amount, 21 percent reported wanting *more* involvement, and only 1 percent wanted *less* involvement. The care partners of black patients and patients in fair-to-poor general health were more likely to feel left out of the decision making (with 34 percent and 29 percent, respectively, reporting they wanted more involvement), as were care partners in the under-forty age group (with 34 percent wanting more involvement). Care partners without a biological or legal relationship to the patient also reported more difficulty establishing a relationship of trust with physicians or other hospital personnel, more difficulty getting information about the patients' care, and less involvement in care and decision making than recognized family members. Of the care partners who were *not* involved in decisions as much as they thought they should be, 89 percent reported that the patients *wanted* them to be involved.

The family's role in decision making has also attracted the attention of medical ethicists. Difficulties in making treatment decisions for the very old and dependent or for patients suffering from dementia have raised ethical and legal issues beyond the scope of this chapter. It is important to note, however, that elderly persons *expect* their families to assume the decision-making role in the event that they are no longer personally able to make health care decisions. Most elderly persons interviewed in one study were comfortable letting family members make such decisions even in the absence of any formalized legal agreements (High, 1988).

Patients and families *want* this involvement. In family practice outpatient settings, patients and family members expressed a desire for family conferences with the physician, to address problems relating to serious illness and behavioral issues (Kushner and others, 1986).

Families take care of sick people. Within the broad spectrum of health care delivery, the largest single provider of care is not the hospital or clinic, the physician or nurse; it is the family (Griffith and Griffith, 1987; Sigmond, 1981). Formal paid providers of home health services account for less than 15 percent of care given to older people in the community; the rest is provided by family members (Freda, 1986). While the caregiving role is not new for families, the demands surrounding it have intensified, as patients are discharged "quicker and sicker" from hospitals and live for years with chronic illness. Families are often unprepared for this responsibility. Both inpatient and outpatient services need to recognize the family's caregiving role and to integrate a family-centered approach into their mission, planning process, and service delivery systems (Fleming, 1987).

Sickness affects the whole family, not just the patient. Patients participating in our focus groups expressed serious concern about the impact of their illness on their families: "My innermost thoughts? My worst fears? 'How is my wife going to react to this? What will it do to her?' Not me— . . . I felt that I would be okay. I was worried, 'what will it do to her?'"

Serious illness often throws families into a crisis that is more serious than the disease itself. Families experience significant emotional, psychosocial, and psychosomatic difficulties. Adding to the physical demands of care is the emotional strain that comes from not knowing if, when, and how the patient will recover. Family members may worry that they will be unequal to the task of caring for the sick person, that they will do the wrong thing, or that they will not have access to the medical resources they need (Brown, Glazer, and Higgins, 1983; Stern and Pascale, 1979; Wishnie, Hackett, and Cassem, 1971). They may blame themselves for the patient's illness, as the wife of a patient having a heart attack reported (Goodman, 1988, p. 48): "I can't help worrying over things I've done, haven't done, should have done, or should have done differently. . . . I am crying and shaking, and finally I throw up. [My husband] is given Demerol, but I feel that I am the one who should be sedated." Sickness may drastically alter usual family roles and behavior patterns, and the needs and expectations of family members may be different from those of the patient (Lewis, 1986). Spouses may worry about the long-term effects of the patient's disability on critical aspects of the marriage relationship, including sexual relations. Families may have to make do without the income that the patient once brought in, while they bear the financial burden of paying for medical care.

The stressful effects of illness on the family may be transient, or they may continue over time and contribute to a deterioration in the health status of family members (Hathaway and others, 1987) or to long-term psychosocial disability (Mayou, Foster, and Williamson, 1978; Northouse, 1988; Stern and Pascale, 1979). Spouses of patients who are seriously ill sometimes show signs of psychosocial disability comparable in frequency, duration, and severity to that experienced by the patients themselves. Reported symptoms include anxiety, depression, fatigue, irritability, poor concentration, and insomnia (Mayou, Foster, and Williamson, 1978).

Chronic psychosocial disability within the family can seriously interfere with the patient's rehabilitation and adjustment, suggesting the need for early intervention to improve coping mechanisms and facilitate family functioning. Family interventions can make a difference, as shown by one study of education and counseling programs for the caregivers of stroke victims (Evans and others, 1988). Education and counseling led to significant improvements both in the caregivers' knowledge and in family functioning at six-month and one-year intervals, when compared to routine follow-up care. Counseling and education together were found to be more effective than education alone, resulting in better patient adjustment and family functioning.

Families influence health behavior, health status and clinical outcomes, and patterns of service utilization. Family involvement in programs of prevention, treatment, and rehabilitation has been demonstrated to speed patients' rate of recovery and lower their risk of mortality, decrease reliance on medical services and lower the rate of rehospitalization, improve patients' adherence to medical regimens, and improve psychosocial and family functioning.

One particularly dramatic study conducted at Johns Hopkins University (Morisky and others, 1983) compared the effectiveness of three different educational interventions—brief individual counseling, instructing the spouse during a home visit, and patient group sessions—on hypertension treatment compliance and overall mortality. While each intervention showed a significant effect, with a 57 percent overall reduction in mortality, the groups that used spouse education tended to do the best, with improved compliance and a significant lowering of patients' blood pressure and mortality.

Chatham (1978) also showed that postcardiotomy patients whose families were taught communication techniques, such as using eye contact, touch, and verbal orientation to time, person, and place, had fewer problems with psychosis than a control group did.

Family support interventions can influence the use of health-related services. The neonatal intensive-care unit at Montreal Children's Hospital developed a family support system designed to increase family involvement and knowledge, identify families at particular risk for psychosocial disability, and improve the continuity of patient care after discharge. During the first two years of the program, 50 percent of children in the control group were rehospitalized, compared to only 31 percent of children whose families had participated in the program. Moreover, the children in the control group visited the emergency room twice as often as those in the study group during the second year of the program, although no significant difference was found during the first year (Perrault and others, 1986).

Seltzer, Ivry, and Litchfield (1987) also found family involvement to influence the utilization of outpatient social services. Family members of elderly persons referred to the Jewish Family and Children's Service in Boston were randomly assigned to an experimental group in which family members were trained in case management skills or to a control group receiving traditional services from the social worker. The essence of the case management approach is to establish a central locus of responsibility for the coordination of services. In the experimental group, family members were viewed as partners with the social worker and had more involvement with coordinating services. In the control group, the social worker was the principal case manager. Families trained as case managers needed, on average, eighty fewer days of service than those in traditional case management programs.

Patients' adherence to medical regimens is strongly influenced by family members' expectations of behavior, and by patients' perceptions of those expectations (McMahon and others, 1986; Miller and others, 1982). Patients whose spouses are supportive are more likely to adhere to their medical regimen (Glasgow and Toobert, 1988), and spouses who believe in the therapeutic benefits of the regimens are more supportive (Doherty, Schrott, Metcalf, and

Iasiello-Vailas, 1983). Showing an interest and reminding the patient to take medication correlate positively with improved compliance; however, nagging about medication or diet has a significant negative correlation with adherence.

The family is a present client and future customer. Most of the patients in our focus groups spoke of their earlier experiences with hospitalized family members—often, an elderly mother or father in declining health. The hospitals that had done well by their parents and supported the family members in those times of family crisis were often the ones that they themselves chose to go to when they became ill. Other hospitals left a correspondingly bad impression and were clearly shunned. From a public relations perspective, then, both the patient and the family are the hospital's clients. Family members make judgments about the quality of care, based on patients' experiences and their own observations. And these judgments influence their own attitudes and future behavior. Institutions that demonstrate their commitment to involve and support families are therefore helping to build their own future constituency.

What Do Families Need?
How Well Are These Needs Met?

Clinicians sometimes dread encounters with patients' family members for fear that their demands will be overwhelming. Just as there are difficult patients who tax the clinicians' patience and time, there are certainly difficult families. Families' expressed needs for information, education, and support are nevertheless reasonable, for the most part justifiable, and often in the patient's best interest. Health care institutions that have made systematic efforts to incorporate patients' families into the care process do not report that this creates an added burden. In fact, difficult families may be less of a problem when they are more involved and when their needs are addressed directly.

In many respects, families want and need the same things patients need—information, understanding, and respect. But families also have some needs that are distinctive and unique to their caregiving role. They may have emotional needs relating to feelings of guilt or issues of dependency and responsibility. They may also need help in caring for the patient. Involving families effectively requires health care providers to recognize both what patients need from their families and what families need for themselves.

Moreover, significant relationships that function as family relationships should be recognized as such. Whatever problems family members report in their relations with hospitals and health professionals, the problem is even more pronounced for "significant others" who are not relatives.

Families need information about the patient's condition and treatment. During the crisis of hospitalization for a serious illness, families place the highest priority on timely, accurate, and honest information about the patient's condition, daily progress, changes in clinical status, and prognosis (Leske, 1986; Molter, 1979; O'Brien, 1983; Rodgers, 1983). And what they complain about most often is lack of information and problems communicating with medical professionals (Molter, 1979; Rodgers, 1983). One family member reported her own anxiety when her husband was hospitalized with an acute myocardial infarction: "The nurses are coming in and out of the cubicle, taking Allan's blood pressure and temperature, adjusting intravenous tubes and oxygen, but nobody tells me what is wrong" (Goodman, 1988, p. 46). Another described a common frustration among families of hospitalized patients: "It was part of a series of communication failures that were growing more frustrating and unnerving by the day. We couldn't reach the doctors by phone or in person unless we caught them during rounds, and the nurses couldn't answer our questions" (DeLeon, 1991, p. 2B).

As these observations suggest, the absence of information and misunderstandings about the patient's condition are a considerable source of anxiety to family members (Mayou, Foster, and Williamson, 1978; Northouse, 1988). In our national survey of recent hospital patients and their care partners, 14 percent of the care partners interviewed felt that they were not given enough information about the patient's condition and medical treatment; 40 percent reported that they were not consulted adequately about the patient's treatment. Twenty-one percent of care partners of patients in public academic health centers did not even know which doctor was in charge.

Families, too, need emotional support. Family members seek out health professionals not only for factual information about the patient's clinical condition, but to reassure themselves that the hospital staff cares about the patient and are providing the best possible care. They also want and need to feel that there is hope. Family members, too, are emotionally vulnerable during the crisis of illness, and yet these needs may fall through the cracks. Among the spouses of terminally ill patients interviewed in one study (Hampe, 1975), 81 percent were informed of their mate's impending death in a hospital hallway or some other public location. Many family members express the need to have a place where they can be alone in the hospital (Molter, 1979; Potter, 1979; Rodgers, 1983) and to have chaplaincy services available (Molter, 1979).

Living with patients with chronic disease or long-term disability also creates distinctive emotional responses and needs among family members. The wife of one focus-group patient who had been hospitalized with a myocardial infarction reluctantly admitted her own continuing fears: "When he's not eating right, and when he's eating things he shouldn't—maybe I shouldn't say these things— I get scared. . . . There were times when it would have been good to talk to someone." The family's worries, in such cases, are likely to be quite different from those of the patient, and they may be reluctant to discuss them in front of patients. In one support group for postoperative cardiac surgical patients at New York University Medical Center, patients and family members initially met together in group sessions. Group leaders discovered, however, that while patients tended to focus on immediate physical symptoms and issues relating to hospitalization, their family members were most concerned about the long-term process of recovery and rehabilitation. Moreover, both patients and families were reticent about emotional issues in each other's presence. Families found it especially hard to deal with patients' anger and depression, while they themselves often felt personally responsible for the patient's recovery. Separate groups for patients and families were then organized, to allow each to give vent to their emotions more openly (Brown, Glazer, and Higgins, 1983). Unfortunately these support groups have been discontinued, but much can still be learned from their experience.

Families need ongoing help with caregiving. When patients

are discharged from the hospital, the primary responsibility for their care shifts away from health care professionals to the families. But families are frequently unprepared for this caregiving role. In our national survey of care partners of hospitalized patients, 24 percent reported having serious worries, most often about their own ability to care for the patient. Yet only 17 percent of the care partners interviewed reported that someone at the hospital discussed their ability to handle things at home after discharge. More than one-third reported that *no one* told them how to help the patient's recovery, 42 percent were not informed about medication side effects, 36 percent were not warned of the danger signals to watch out for, and nearly one-third received no dietary advice or instructions (see Table 8.1). Interview responses also suggested that many health professionals spend too little time discussing home care with family members: over one-third of the care partners interviewed said that doctors and nurses spent *no time at all* discussing such matters prior to discharge (see Table 8.2).

The long-term responsibility of caring for sick relatives may require family members to learn new caregiving skills. They also need to know about available services and resources, how to coordinate these services, and how to navigate through the health care system. And they need to find ways to cope with the ongoing stress of illness. Interventions that help families adjust to the demands of caregiving can enhance their role as a partner in patient-centered care. Families of multiple sclerosis patients, for example, have demonstrated an improved ability to deal constructively with the disability when they understand the illness, develop mechanisms for coping with it, and participate in support services (Power, 1985). Families of cancer patients at home similarly express the need for help with various aspects of continuous caregiving: help in understanding the illness and what to expect; help in managing diet (Northouse, 1988), giving chemotherapy injections, and managing side effects; help in reassuring the patients and giving them hope; help managing the household and finances, amid the added burden of illness; and help with the emotional strain that comes from "standing by" while a loved one suffers (Stetz, 1987).

Families of patients with chronic illness also need relief from the twenty-four-hour-per-day demands of providing care in the

Table 8.1. Involvement of Care Partners in Discharge Planning, Picker/Commonwealth National Survey.

	How and when to take medication (percent)	Medication side effects (percent)	Diet recommendations (percent)	Activity recommendations (percent)	When to resume normal activities (percent)	When to return to work (percent)	Danger signals of illness (percent)	How to help recovery (percent)
				Were you told?				
Told	74	55	58	72	66	38	58	61
Not told	16	42	30	23	29	21	36	34
Does not apply	9		11	5	4	41	5	4
Not sure	1	3	1	1	1	1	1	1

Table 8.2. Involvement of Care Partners in Posthospital
Care/Discharge Planning, Picker/Commonwealth National Survey.

	Minutes of discussion of what to do at home		
	By doctor (percent)	By nurse (percent)	By social worker (percent)
No time	34	36	82
5 minutes or less	13	15	3
5–15 minutes	31	29	5
15+ minutes	20	17	6
Not sure	3	3	3

home. In spite of their strong need for respite care and assistance in the home, families are often unaware of the support services that exist or of how they can gain access to them (Caserta, Lund, Wright, and Redburn, 1987; Lewis, 1986).

What Can Hospitals Do to Involve Families and Meet Their Needs?

Some interventions hospitals have developed to involve families more actively in patient care require a radical restructuring of health care services; others more modestly target specific needs. All of them, however, advance the overall goal of enhancing patient-centered care. We discuss these interventions in terms of three defined roles for families and "significant others": caregiver or care partner, health promoter, and source of emotional support. However, these categories are not mutually exclusive, and many examples of successful programs overlap two or more.

Involve family or friends as caregivers or care partners. Caregiver programs are designed to enhance the family's ability to provide direct assistance in meeting the patient's basic health care needs. As the daughter of a patient with gallbladder disease observed, "It might be helpful if the nurses could encourage relatives to do very simple caring tasks like brushing someone's hair or washing someone's hands" (Wertheimer, 1987, p. 28). Using the family as a health care resource is not an innovative idea. Its roots lie in traditional medicine, and it has been practiced in other cultures for centuries. However, the renewed emphasis on the family's role in medicine reflects an attempt to recapture the warm and caring quality that high-technology Western medicine may have lost and to prepare families to take care of patients with chronic illness.

One particularly successful application of this focus on a return to traditional family values has been the rise of the birthing center and family-oriented maternity care. Birthing centers, which gained popularity in the early 1970s, were established in response to child-bearing women's expressed desire to experience labor and deliver in a homelike atmosphere, to exercise control over their own bodies and choices about their medical treatment, and to remain in touch with loved ones during hospitalization (Timberlake, 1975). This family orientation extended to arrangements permitting infants to "room in" with the mother and siblings to visit the hospital to help smooth the transition of mother and new baby to home after discharge (Renaud, 1981). The popularity of birthing centers, whether as a separate facility or within the hospital maternity service, provides an example of how changes in consumer attitudes can successfully drive changes in service delivery (Allgaier, 1978).

Cooperative care is another model program that emphasizes patient and family education and responsibility in the hospital setting (Grieco and others, 1990). The prototype is New York University Medical Center's 120-bed Cooperative Care Unit, which has been in operation since 1979. Patients admitted to the unit must be stable, but they need not be ambulatory. Each must be accompanied by a friend or family member who serves as a care partner. As a rule, but not always, care partners are expected to spend the night. They are taught what signs and symptoms to look out for and are instructed, along with the patients, in whatever routines the patients are expected to carry out on their own, in the hospital or at home. While the patients are in the hospital, however, care partners are not expected to take the place of nurses in performing such tasks as taking and charting vital signs or changing dressings, unless these activities are part of the patients' home care. Their primary function, instead, is to serve both as supportive companions and as "eyes and ears" for the medical staff. Together, patient and care partner are accommodated in hotel-like double rooms free of such high-tech trappings as central suction, oxygen, or monitoring equipment. Nursing stations, treatment and examination rooms, and clinical consultation areas are physically separate, located on a different floor entirely. Meals, too, are taken in a central, communal dining room, where patients select food cafeteria style. Nurses, freed from housekeeping and routine custodial nursing chores, play a more active role in educating patients and care partners to care for themselves at home. A formal evaluation of Coop Care conducted under the auspices of the Health Care Financing Administration concluded that it was an appropriate and less costly alternative for patients with an underlying chronic condition (Levine and others, 1987). The evidence gathered also suggested that Coop Care patients did better than the control group at long-term compliance with regimens requiring changes in entrenched behaviors (such as smoking cessation and diet changes), most likely because of the involvement of their care partners.

From the hospital's perspective, too, the reliance on care partners is one of the unit's strongest points. Not only is it one of the biggest sources of cost savings on the unit, because of the need for less intensive staffing, but supporters claim it is far superior to the usual methods of keeping patients under surveillance. Liability, an early concern of Coop Care's planners, has not been a problem, probably because care partners are good observers, and the self-administered-medication program eliminates the "wrong-patient" type of medication errors that are fairly common elsewhere. But arranging for a care partner can be difficult for patients, given travel time and the competing demands of jobs, family, and children. Moreover, patients are much more likely to take out their hostilities and anxieties on friends or family members than they are on staff, and while this may be understandable for the patients, it is hard on their care partners. Burnout is a real hazard. This model of care is not for everyone. The payoff for care partners, however, is that they are much better equipped to take care of the patients when they go home.

In a German rehabilitation unit for patients with head injuries, family members stay in the room with the patient and assist with simple nursing care. The room is furnished with objects familiar to the patient, such as pictures from home, cassettes of the patient's favorite music, and souvenirs. The staff was impressed with how quickly the patient became reoriented and how quickly the patient's restlessness and irritability resolved. As the patient improves, the rooming-in arrangement is stopped to encourage a return to independence (Date, Goede, and Werner, 1987).

The "Family as Team Members" Program at Harmarville Rehabilitation Center in Pittsburgh, Pennsylvania, involves families of stroke patients in the rehabilitation process throughout hospitalization. Families receive information on classes and support groups and a videotape presentation that emphasizes their importance as a member of the rehabilitation team. Throughout the hospital stay, families have opportunities to observe the patient's therapy and care; to meet with members of the rehabilitation team, including physicians; and to assist the patient with exercise, diet, physical care, and other activities of daily living. Other resources available to the family include a "how-to" book for dealing with common problems relating to stroke (Fleming, 1987).

The home care program at M. D. Anderson Hospital in Houston, Texas, was developed to facilitate the transition from hospital to home. Informal one-to-one teaching begins on admission, followed by educational classes on home chemotherapy and general home care. Volunteers personally invite the family members to participate, accompany them to class, and act as a link between the family and staff. The program is also promoted through brochures and videotapes that are played in the hospital cafeteria and waiting rooms (Fleming, 1987).

El Camino Hospital's Project Transition in Mountain View, California, works with families of patients at high risk for rehospitalization to ease the transition from hospital to home. Trained volunteers visit the patient and family at home on the day of discharge to provide emotional support and assist with unanticipated home care needs, including grocery shopping, respite care, obtaining prescription medication, coordinating home care services or equipment, providing information on community resources, or running errands. The volunteer will continue to telephone the patient and family during the week following discharge to answer questions and to offer assistance (Fleming, 1987).

Texas Children's Hospital's cystic fibrosis program for parents has four educational components: (1) discharge preparation teaching during hospitalization, (2) a series of five classes after discharge for parents of newly diagnosed children to provide information on the disease and training in management skills, (3) support groups for parents, and (4) a continuing series of informational meetings on special topics. The program is structured to meet the changing informational needs of the caregiver at various stages of chronic illness (Fleming, 1987).

The Education and Family Support Services at the Neurological Sciences Center of the Good Samaritan Hospital and Medical Center in Portland, Oregon, is an impressive example of a comprehensive program designed to meet the variety of needs of caregivers of neurological patients. Designed initially to serve the hospital's inpatient clinical services, the program was later expanded to include a wide variety of outpatient programs and services targeting the unmet needs of caregivers in the community (Fleming, 1987). Program components include the following: (1) "Helping You Care," a five-week class for caregivers, which was developed in collaboration with the American Red Cross; (2) a lecture series for caregivers; (3) support groups for caregivers; (4) a training program for peer counselors; (5) an advocacy group for neurological patients; (6) a respite care program; (7) a legal and financial planning class; (8) a resource center, which provides public information on neurological problems and caregiving issues; (9) classes on specific neurological diseases, such as Alzheimer's; (10) public education videotapes; (11) and handbooks and training manuals for caregivers (Heagarty, Dunn, and Watson, 1988). The program encourages physicians to refer patients to the Education and Family Support Services by distributing a "prescription pad" with a checklist of available services.

Recognize friends or family as health promoters. Recognizing that patients' health-related behaviors and habits are strongly influenced by their family and social circles, many health promotion programs try to help families encourage and support patients' efforts to adopt healthier life-styles. If patients need to alter their diet, for example, the family members who plan the menus, shop for food, and prepare the meals will also need nutrition education.

Many hospitals now involve family members in the cardiac rehabilitation process and give families the same instructions regarding life-style changes that they give to patients (Biegel, Sales, and Schultz, 1991). Four Southern California cardiac rehabilitation centers have developed a model program, which includes ten 90-minute group sessions for patients and their spouses conducted by a cardiovascular rehabilitation nurse and psychiatric nurse. The group sessions are designed to offer support to spouses, to involve them in the process of changing life-style and behavior, and to help them clarify their role and avoid the pitfalls of becoming "watchdogs" (Dracup, Meleis, Baker, and Edlefsen, 1984).

Help friends and family members to provide patients with emotional support. A family's ability to provide the emotional support patients need and rely on may be compromised by the fragility of their own coping mechanisms, under the stress of illness. Families, then, no less than patients, need emotional support to cope with illness. Programs that offer assistance and support to families can help relieve their anxiety and help them cope. Such programs may vary in format and structure and in the specific emotional needs they address. Some groups are organized specifically to offer emotional support to families in similar circumstances. Many educational and social support programs also include an emotional support component. Among the recurring issues they address are family members' need for catharsis and feelings and expressions of depression and anger, family members' loss of the sense of well-being, problems of communication with the patient and with medical staff, fears of death, issues relating to employment and work, apprehension about discharge and rehabilitation, and fears about sexual performance and behavior (Harding and Morefield, 1976).

Family members often feel cast in the role of watchdogs whose job it is to force patients to comply with prescribed treatment regimens. While they play an important role in supporting needed behavior change, the nagging watchdog image can have a negative effect on their personal relationships. Cardiac rehabilitation programs at Valley Regional Hospital in Claremont, New Hampshire (Fleming, 1987), and New York University Medical Center (Brown, Glazer, and Higgins, 1983) are examples of programs that offer families assistance in handling these conflicts. These support groups address how to deal with noncompliance and be supportive without nagging. A pain control intervention at Memorial Medical Center, Long Beach, California, similarly helps patients and families of persons living with chronic pain to alleviate the dominating effect of pain on the patient's life by helping them identify, and avoid reinforcing, negative behaviors (Fleming, 1987). This in-hospital intervention includes the family component so that family members will understand their role in pain control and what they can do to help. According to the staff psychologist, patients, families, and staff view this program very positively.

A number of interventions have also been developed to provide families with support and information when patients are hospitalized in intensive care units. The Family Crisis Intervention Program at University Hospital in Columbus, Ohio, is one example. It includes the following components: (1) a family assessment questionnaire kept at the patient's bedside to help nurses gather appropriate information about the family; (2) a "Telefamily Program," which designates a staff nurse to call a designated family member daily to provide updated information; (3) family orientation to the intensive care unit; (4) the use of volunteers to provide information and emotional support to families in the waiting room (Hodovanic, Reardon, Reese, and Hedges, 1984). This program has also started using a family beeper program on a limited basis. While this program is demanding in terms of nursing time, the nursing staff report that they enjoy the emotional payoff they get from the program. Other programs, including "Intensive Care for Relatives" at Washoe Medical Center in Reno, Nevada (Hoover, 1979), and at UCLA Medical Center's coronary care unit (Breu and Dracup, 1978), similarly aim to address the emotional and informational needs of families systematically.

A simple, low-cost intervention was developed at Riverside

Medical Center, Kankakee, Illinois, by inviting family members to write their goals and expectations of the patient's rehabilitation program into the patient care plan. A nurse reviews the family's comments to identify points of compatibility and mismatch between the family's and the staff's expectations (Fleming, 1987).

At Pilgrim Psychiatric Center on Long Island, New York, a lack of communication between the family members and staff was identified as a problem. The center responded by increasing staff availability on evenings, when most family members visited. Families were also mailed information about dates and times that team members could be consulted. This simple change significantly improved family participation in treatment planning (Carbonara, 1980). In addition, once a month, families meet with staff in a family forum to discuss a variety of issues.

Providing even simple sleeping accommodations for family members of hospitalized patients can make it easier for them to stay physically close to the patients at critical times. The Planetree Model Unit at California Pacific Medical Center in San Francisco allows families to visit twenty-four hours a day and makes cots and sleeping couches available to those who want to stay overnight. This "rooming-in" approach is also used extensively in many pediatric hospital wards, with beds, cots, or fold-down chairs available to parents in the patient's room or in lounge areas. St. Marys Hospital in Rochester, Minnesota, also permits family members to stay overnight in its transitional care unit, converted from an unused hospital ward. Other hospitals have arranged accommodations for family members, especially those traveling from some distance, nearby but off site. The Ronald McDonald houses are famous for providing accommodations and support to the parents of very sick children in a homelike atmosphere near numerous pediatric hospitals. Other hospitals, such as M. D. Anderson in Houston, Texas, have made arrangements with nearby hotels to accommodate families and to provide support services at the hotel.

Planned recreational activities for families of sick patients can offer welcome diversions and create opportunities for emotional support. Harper-Grace Hospitals in Detroit, Michigan, offer families of cancer patients weekend retreats in a wooded setting, where they can explore ways of coping with the disease. Group discussions, formal presentations, and art and music activities offer families verbal and nonverbal channels of communication and encourage the expression of feeling. Specially designed activities, such as a puppet show that invites audience participation, permit children to express their concerns (Fleming, 1987). Both family members and staff have described this upbeat program as an uplifting and positive experience.

M. D. Anderson Hospital in Houston, Texas, has also designed programs and activities especially for the families of pediatric cancer patients, including siblings. The hospital-sponsored Camp Star Trails provides a normal camp experience for children with cancer and their siblings. The hospital also provides individual counseling for patients and siblings with a "child life worker" (Fleming, 1987).

Summary

Patient-centered care is also family-centered care. Bearing this in mind, providers can begin to address their patients' needs more effectively if they ask themselves the following questions:

- Are families receiving adequate information? Are they included in educational programs and processes?
- Are families allowed and encouraged, whenever possible, to participate in care? Are they trained in appropriate caregiving skills?
- Are families involved and included in discharge plans?
- Do families understand how their life-style and behaviors affect health? Do they understand how to change their behavior?
- Does the hospital make systematic efforts to help relieve the anxiety of family members and help them cope with the stress of illness?

We have briefly outlined a variety of interventions that have been developed in different institutional settings to address families' needs. We present these programs not as solutions, but rather as a guide to help managers come up with creative approaches suited to their own institutions.

Suggestions for Improvement

- Schedule regular times, convenient to most families, when staff will be available to counsel, educate, or meet with designated family members, and inform families in writing of those dates and times.
- Encourage family members to write down or express their own goals and expectations for the patient's care, and include these family notes in the patient's chart or at the bedside, where staff can read them.
- Provide bulletin boards at the bedside where patients and family members can post questions or comments.
- Offer patients and their families written or videotaped take-home materials with health information appropriate to their needs.
- Develop an order form or "prescription pad" for physicians and other providers, with a checklist of available family support and referral services.
- Train volunteers to serve as liaison between staff and families in waiting rooms outside emergency rooms, operating rooms, or intensive care units; these volunteers should keep the family informed about the patient's progress, how long the wait will be, what to expect, and so on, and help them locate needed services and accommodations.
- Allow and encourage family members to help with the patient's personal and nonmedical care wherever possible, including wheeling them to x-ray and helping with bathing, eating, and other activities of daily living.
- Offer a nonalcoholic "Happy Hour" or other social occasion for patients and family members, to help them establish their own informal support network.
- Train volunteers to visit the patient and family at home soon after discharge to help with unanticipated home care needs, such as

filling prescriptions, running errands, coordinating home care services, or providing referrals to community resources.

- Develop a family assessment form to use at the patient's bedside to help providers gather pertinent information and assess the family's needs.

- Include patients and family members on committees and task forces to plan or evaluate services, including patient education and discharge planning.

- Make family involvement and support an explicit part of the organizational mission.

References

Allgaier, A. "Alternative Birth Centers Offer Family-Centered Care." *Hospitals,* 1978, *52,* 97–112.

Biegel, D. E., Sales, E., and Schultz, R. *Family Caregiving in Chronic Illness.* Newbury Park, Calif.: Sage, 1991.

Breu, C., and Dracup, K. "Helping the Spouses of Critically Ill Patients." *American Journal of Nursing,* 1978, *78*(1), 51–53.

Brown, D. G., Glazer, H., and Higgins, M. "Group Intervention: A Psychosocial and Educational Approach to Open Heart Surgery Patients and Their Families." *Social Work in Health Care,* 1983, *9*(2), 47–59.

Carbonara, D. P. "Family Visits and Involvement in Treatment of Patients at a State Hospital." *Hospital and Community Psychiatry,* 1980, *31*(12), 854–855.

Caserta, M. S., Lund, D. A., Wright, S. D., and Redburn, D. E. "Caregivers to Dementia Patients: The Utilization of Community Services." *Gerontologist,* 1987, *27*(2), 209–214.

Chatham, M. A. "The Effect of Family Involvement on Patients' Manifestations of Post-Cardiotomy Psychosis." *Heart and Lung,* 1978, *7*(6), 995–999.

Darbyshire, P. "Sour Grapes." *Nursing Times,* 1987, *83*(37), 23–25.

Date, E., Goede, G., and Werner, G. "Familiar Faces." *Nursing Times,* 1987, *83*(37), 26–27.

DeLeon, C. "Patience: No Pain, No Gain." *Philadelphia Inquirer,* May 5, 1991, p. 2B.

Doherty, W. J., Schrott, H. G., Metcalf, L., and Iasiello-Vailas, L. "Effect of Spouse Support and Health Beliefs on Medication Adherence." *Journal of Family Practice*, 1983, *17*(5), 837–841.

Dracup, K., Meleis, A., Baker, K., and Edlefsen, P. "Family-Focused Cardiac Rehabilitation—A Role Supplementation Program for Cardiac Patients and Spouses." *Nursing Clinics of North America*, 1984, *19*(1), 113–124.

Evans, R. L., and others. "Family Intervention After Stroke: Does Counseling or Education Help?" *Stroke*, 1988, *19*(10), 1243.

Fleming, S. "Supporting the Family's Role in Patient Recovery, Rehabilitation." *Promoting Health*, 1987, *8* (Supplement), 1–12.

Freda, K. "Supporting Family Caregiving." *Iowa Medicine*, 1986, *76*(10), 466–468.

Glasgow, R. E., and Toobert, D. J. "Social Environment and Regimen Adherence Among Type II Diabetic Patients." *Diabetes Care*, 1988, *11*(5), 377–386.

Goodman, E. J. "Without Warning: Diary of a Heart Attack." *New York*, 1988, *21*, 44–51.

Grieco, A. J., and others. "New York University Medical Center's Cooperative Care Unit: Patient Education and Family Participation During the Hospitalization—The First Ten Years." *Patient Education and Counseling*, 1990, *15*, 3–15.

Griffith, J. L., and Griffith, M. E. "Structural Family Therapy in Chronic Illness." *Psychosomatics*, 1987, *28*(4), 202–205.

Hampe, S. O. "Needs of the Grieving Spouse in a Hospital Setting." *Nursing Research*, 1975, *24*(2), 113–119.

Harding, A. L., and Morefield, M. "Group Interventions for Wives of Myocardial Infarction Patients." *Nursing Clinics of North America*, 1976, *11*, 339–347.

Hathaway, D., and others. "Health Promotion and Disease Prevention for the Hospitalized Patient's Family." *Nurse Administration Quarterly*, 1987, *11*(3), 1–7.

Heagarty, B., Dunn, L., and Watson, M. A. "They Are Not Alone: Lending Support to Family Caregivers." *Health Progress*, 1988, *69*(11), 55–58, 75.

High, D. M. "All in the Family: Extended Autonomy and Expectations in Surrogate Health Care Decision-Making." *Gerontologist,* 1988, *28* (Supplement), 46–51.

Hodovanic, B. H., Reardon, D., Reese, W., and Hedges, B. "Family Crisis Intervention Program in the Medical Intensive Care Unit." *Heart & Lung,* 1984, *13*(3), 243–249.

Hoover, M. J. "Intensive Care for Relatives." *Hospitals,* 1979, *53,* 219–222.

Kushner, K., and others. "The Family Conference: What Do Patients Want?" *Journal of Family Practice,* 1986, *23*(5), 463–467.

Leske, J. S. "Needs of Relatives of Critically Ill Patients: A Follow-Up." *Heart & Lung,* 1986, *15*(2), 189–193.

Levine, D. M., and others. *Prevention of Future Utilization of Health and Long Term Service Study.* Baltimore: Center for Health Services Research and Development and the Division of Internal Medicine, Johns Hopkins University, 1987.

Lewis, F. M. "The Impact of Cancer on the Family: A Critical Analysis of the Research Literature." *Patient Education and Counseling,* 1986, *8*(3), 269–289.

McMahon, M., and others. "Life Situations, Health Beliefs, and Medical Regimen Adherence of Patients with Myocardial Infarction." *Heart & Lung,* 1986, *15*(1), 82–86.

Mayou, R., Foster, A., and Williamson, B. "The Psychological and Social Effects of Myocardial Infarction on Wives." *British Medical Journal,* 1978, *18,* 699–701.

Miller, P., and others. "Health Beliefs of and Adherence to the Medical Regimen by Patients with Ischemic Heart Disease." *Heart & Lung,* 1982, *11*(4), 332–339.

Molter, N. C. "Needs of Relatives of Critically Ill Patients: A Descriptive Study." *Heart & Lung,* 1979, *8*(2), 332–339.

Morisky, D. E., and others. "Five-Year Blood Pressure Control and Mortality Following Health Education for Hypertensive Patients." *American Journal of Public Health,* 1983, *73,* 153–162.

Northouse, L. L. "Family Issues in Cancer Care. *Advances in Psychosomatic Medicine,* 1988, *18,* 82–101.

O'Brien, M. E. "An Identification of the Needs of Family Members of Terminally Ill Patients in a Hospital Setting." *Military Medicine,* 1983, *148,* 712–716.

Perrault, C., and others. "Family Support System in Newborn Medicine: Does It Work? Follow-Up Study of Infants at Risk." *Journal of Pediatrics*, 1986, *108*(6), 1025-1030.

Potter, P. A. "Stress and the Intensive Care Unit—The Family's Perception." *Missouri Nursing*, 1979, *48*, 5-8.

Power, P. W. "Family Coping Behaviors in Chronic Illness: A Rehabilitation Perspective." *Rehabilitation Literature*, 1985, *46*(3, 4), 78-83.

Renaud, M. "Parental Response to Family-Centered Maternity Care and to Implementation of Sibling Visits." *Military Medicine*, 1981, *146*, 850-852.

Rodgers, C. D. "Needs of Relatives of Cardiac Surgery Patients During the Critical Care Phase." *Focus on Critical Care*, 1983, *19*(5), 50-55.

Rosenbaum, E. E. *The Doctor.* New York: Ballantine Books, 1988.

Seltzer, M. M., Ivry, J., and Litchfield, L. C. "Family Members as Case Managers: Partnership Between the Formal and Informal Support Networks." *Gerontologist*, 1987, *27*(6), 722-728.

Sigmond, R. M. "Hospital Planning Should Provide for Family Role in Care." *Hospitals*, 1981, *55*(12), 63-64, 113.

Stern, M. J., and Pascale, L. "Psychosocial Adaptation Post-Myocardial Infarction: The Spouse's Dilemma." *Journal of Psychosomatic Research*, 1979, *23*, 83-87.

Stetz, K. M. "Caregiving Demands During Advanced Cancer—The Spouse's Needs." *Cancer Nursing*, 1987, *10*(5), 260-268.

Timberlake, B. "The New Life Center." *American Journal of Nursing*, 1975, *75*(9), 1456-1461.

Wertheimer, A. "Just Visiting." *Nursing Times*, 1987, *83*(37), 28-29.

Wishnie, H. A., Hackett, T. P., and Cassem, N. "Psychological Hazards of Convalescence Following Myocardial Infarction." *Journal of the American Medical Association*, 1971, *215*(8), 1292-1296.

9

Facilitating the Transition Out of the Hospital

Beth Ellers
Janice D. Walker

While they are in the hospital, patients exist in a self-contained, sequestered environment. Hospital personnel who can meet most of their daily needs are only a call-button away. But many patients worry about how they will take care of themselves, about whether they will be able to restore their health and lead a normal life after they leave the hospital. A "jump-off into nowhere," one patient described it; a "jump-off into uncharted territory . . . away from this warm and cozy environment." The anxiety that such a "jump-off" can provoke can be considerable, as Edward Rosenbaum's thoughts about his own impending discharge in *The Doctor* suggest: "'Go home?' I thought. They gave me a general anesthetic, they cut my throat, and they haven't even given me a drink. Now they're sending me home? What if I can't swallow? What if I start to bleed? What if my throat swells in the middle of the night and I can't catch my breath?" (1988, p. 42). From the perspective of patients, hospitalization is an episode in a continuum of illness experience. Their concerns reflect the broader perspective of how illness impacts on their lives.

This dimension of patient-centered care has been thought of traditionally as *discharge planning*. However, to better integrate the hospital experience into patients' lives, hospitals should shift the emphasis from *getting patients out* of the hospital to *facilitating the transition*. Discharge planning too often calls to mind a list of

204

instructions given to patients five minutes before they leave the hospital. We broaden the definition to include the process of hospital-related activities that involve the patient, the family, and health care providers working together to facilitate the transition from one environment to another. According to Shine (1983), this "transition and continuity" dimension of care includes a systematic, multilevel process:

- Assessing patients' resources and limitations during hospitalization to determine their needs
- Providing patients with the education necessary to care for themselves at home
- Counseling patients to facilitate the stressful transition between hospital and home, dependence and independence
- Planning for continuity in health care on discharge from the hospital
- Coordinating individual, family, hospital, and community resources needed to implement the plan for this transition
- Following up at home to determine the effectiveness of the discharge plan and to assess changes in need

Health care professionals want to improve this transition process. In 1987, a national panel of medical and quality assurance experts met to select potential topics for advancing routine quality assurance work for older patients. Of the twenty-seven health care services rated by these experts, none received higher ratings for importance, frequency of use, or feasibility of measuring effectiveness than did hospital discharge planning. The experts gave discharge planning the highest possible score for patient benefit, the lowest possible score for current quality, and the highest score for improvability (Fink and others, 1987).

Studies have shown that both hospitals and patients benefit from facilitating the transition out of the hospital. The evidence suggests that such benefits include the following: improved patient outcomes (Rubenstein and others, 1984), increased patient satisfaction (Berkman and others, 1988), decreased length of hospital stay (Barker and others, 1985; Cunningham, 1981; Kennedy, Neidlinger, and Scroggins, 1987; Schwartz, Blumenfield, and Simon, 1990), fewer hospital readmissions (Naylor, 1990; Rubenstein and others, 1984), enhanced cost-effectiveness (Safran and Phillips, 1989; Weinberger, Smith, Katz, and Moore, 1988), and lower mortality (Rubenstein and others, 1984).

While humanitarian concern for patients is reason enough to justify improvements in transition planning, the expense of *not* addressing these issues can burden the health care system financially. In an analysis of Medicare expenditures, 22 percent of Medicare hospitalizations were followed by readmissions within sixty days of discharge; readmissions accounted for 24 percent of Medicare inpatient expenditures (Anderson and Steinberg, 1984). It is estimated that 59 percent of unplanned hospital readmissions in one study were avoidable (Williams and Fitton, 1988).

Numerous discharge planning studies have focused on decreasing hospital length of stay and readmissions (Barker and others, 1985; Berkman and Abrams, 1986; Berkman and others, 1988; Cunningham, 1981; Kennedy, Neidlinger, and Scroggins, 1987; McPhee and others, 1983; Naylor, 1990; Safran and Phillips, 1989; Saltz and others, 1988; Smith, Weinberger, Katz, and Moore, 1988; Weinberger, Smith, Katz, and Moore, 1988). While the findings of these studies have been inconsistent, comprehensive planning programs for post-hospital care do show promise in improving patient outcomes in ways that are beneficial for both patients and hospitals.

Facilitating the transition out of the hospital has the added benefit of focusing the care on the patient rather than on the hospital. The patient-centered approach incorporates the patient's short-term and long-term health care needs into the transition process.

The patients we have talked to have been eloquent in describing the importance of a smooth transition from the hospital to home, and hospitals have been inventive in finding ways to ease the passage. This chapter focuses on the patients' view of this process and potential approaches to improving it. These approaches range from a conceptual framework for examining transitional issues to practical interventions that hospitals have used to assist their patients with this transition.

The Patient's Perspective: Problems and Interventions

Patients report they are not receiving adequate clinical information during hospitalization to make the transition to the community. "I got no counseling at all from the university [hospital]. All I got from the university was some pamphlets—about sex, was one." Patients need information on treatment regimens, the clinical course of their illness, and life-style modification on discharge from the hospital. Frequently, however, they either do not receive or do not remember this information and have difficulty following the home care plan. In our Picker/Commonwealth survey of hospital patients discharged to the community (the survey excluded patients discharged to nursing homes or other alternative care facilities), nearly one-third (30 percent) reported not being told about medication side effects. More than one-third (36 percent) said they were not told what foods they could or could not eat. Many patients reported not being told about what danger signals related to their illness to watch for, when to resume normal activities, when to return to work, or how to help their recovery (Walker, 1991).

In another study (Jones, Densen, and Brown, 1989), 64 percent of patients said no one in the hospital had talked with them about managing at home. These findings echo results of a study in which Lindenberg and Coulton (1980) interviewed patients one month after discharge from the hospital about their need for home medical and nursing care and assistance with activities of daily living. Fewer than 60 percent of the patients felt their needs were being adequately met. These findings confirm the need for rethinking the transition planning process to ensure that patients leave the hospital with adequate information to follow their treatment regimen and a healthy life-style.

Why do patients not get adequate information? Either no one is telling them, or they are being told but do not remember. If patients are not getting the information, the explanation may be a combination of time constraints of overburdened health care staff and confusion about who is or should be providing this information. The role of the physician, the nurse, and the social worker in planning for posthospital care is often not clearly defined. Confusion over these responsibilities can also lead to "turf battles." Patients often look to their physician for clinical information, but the physician may have limited time. Perhaps patients are told the information but do not remember it. The stresses of illness and hospitalization can impair the memory or the learning process. This suggests the importance of providing education and reinforcement of the message before, during, and after hospitalization.

To help get more information to patients at Thomas Jefferson University Hospital in Philadelphia, the pharmacy and nursing departments co-developed medication teaching cards as educational aids used in discharge counseling for cardiac patients. These cards are included in the discharge packet and may be tailored to the individual patient's needs by adding specific written instructions (McGinty, Chase, and Mercer, 1988). Patients at Jackson-Madison County General Hospital leave the hospital with a copy of their discharge summary, including instructions for home care (Campbell, 1991). The use of educational aids to reinforce the clinical information assists the patient in following the treatment regimen.

The Learning Center at the University of Minnesota Hospital and Clinic in Minneapolis is designed to teach patients and their families high-tech health-related activities in preparation for discharge. The center is a "lab-like environment" for learning and practicing skills with mannequins and real medical equipment. Patients and family members receive training in such skills as giving injections, managing parenteral nutrition, and caring for central venous catheters (Sumpmann, 1989), ensuring they have adequate technical skills to manage posthospital care. Life-style modification educational programs are also critical to provide patients with the information and ability to change health-related behaviors.

Patients report that their emotional and psychosocial needs are not adequately addressed. As one patient told us, "There is a big disparity between the amount of TLC you get in the hospital and when you're discharged and you go home. You're on your own, baby. I think for people who are insecure, having had a heart attack, . . . every little twinge and every little ache, you figure . . . this is it, baby."

Hospitalization and illness precipitate an emotional crisis for patients and their families. Homecoming may result in concerns about one's illness, disability, loss of control, and dependency. Patients fear that they may have difficulty resuming a "normal" life-style. Roles within the family may undergo upheaval. Fears about potential inability to work and financial burdens may be overwhelming to the patient and family. For patients transferred to an alternative care facility instead of the expected return to home, the emotional issues may be highly charged.

Some patients may not be ready to confront the difficulties of posthospital care while they are in the hospital, but they still need access to services after they are discharged: "I don't think I was prepared for how I felt after the surgery. Part of it was my fault. I was anxious to get out of the hospital, and I had them just give me a staple remover. . . . I didn't appreciate how really wiped out I would be for weeks afterward." Twenty percent of the patients we surveyed nationally reported having serious worries about difficulties they would have after leaving the hospital, and nearly half of these (42 percent) said *no one at the hospital helped with these issues*. They most often worried about how they would care for themselves, the effectiveness of their treatment, whether they would suffer a relapse, and how they would live with their condition (Walker, 1991).

Frequently, patients are more concerned with the impact of the illness on their lives than with the pathophysiology of the disease. The psychosocial sequelae of illness are often the most significant factors of the illness to the patient and the family and can be significant determinants of the patient's adherence to treatment regimens, recovery, and general well-being. Hospitals must not ignore this critical component of posthospital care in their transition planning processes.

Patients often want more control and choice in posthospital care. Health care providers often view discharge planning as "something done *by* professionals *for* patients" (Coulton, Dunkle, Goode, and MacIntosh, 1982). Such one-sided activity may result in giving a list of instructions to the patients as they are wheeled out the door, or researching options and making long-term care plans without consulting the patients. Or only one option may be offered. The elderly, in particular, may feel that decisions are made for them by others (Dubler, 1988). Elderly patients who have been more involved in decision making, on the other hand, have been more satisfied with the outcome of the discharge planning process (Coulton, Dunkle, Goode, and MacIntosh, 1982). Planning for posthospital care should be an *interactive* process with a patient-centered focus. Involving the patient in planning for posthospital care enhances the learning process and improves adherence to medical regimens (Bailey and others, 1987).

Patient participation in decision making about posthospital care influences well-being, health status, and even mortality rates (Abramson, 1990). Abramson outlines practice patterns that support patient autonomy, including the following: (1) involving patients and families together, (2) addressing conflicts that may interfere with patient choice or active participation in decision making, (3) creating a sense of choice through a discussion of available options, (4) preparing the patient for discharge emotionally as well as logistically, and (5) encouraging others involved in the patient's care to promote patient autonomy.

The first step in preparing some patients for discharge is to encourage them to ask for help and to be advocates for their own health care. Patients may be afraid to ask for help or may not recognize the hospital as an appropriate resource for assistance with home care. One way of addressing this issue is to show patients a videotape about preparing for the posthospital transition. By portraying specific examples of problems patients often encounter following hospitalization, the tape can help them understand what to expect and encourage their involvement. The tape also can provide information about resources available to assist them with their concerns about discharge and home care.

A simple intervention to encourage patient involvement in planning is to require patients to write down their questions prior to discharge. These questions should be discussed at a discharge interview conducted by the patient's physician, nurse, or social worker, and the patient should not be discharged until needs and concerns for posthospital care are addressed.

Cooperative Care at New York University Hospital focuses on enhanced patient and family participation through creation of a homelike environment that mimics the "real world." Patients administer their own medications, after they have been properly trained by a pharmacist, and they select their own meals at a cafeteria-style dining center. Pharmacy, nutrition, and nursing staff are available to address the patient's and family's educational needs and to promote healthy behaviors, but the *responsibility* rests with the patient. This expanded participation facilitates the transition to home, because the patient and family are encouraged to "practice" health-related activities and behaviors in a setting that emphasizes education.

Patients can also get information from resources outside the hospital. M. D. Anderson Hospital in Houston, Texas, provides a network of former patients and their family members to assist patients and families in their geographical location. For Texas and Western Louisiana, M. D. Anderson also offers a Telephone Information Service (1-800-4-CANCER), which provides a directory of community resources in the geographical area. This service was developed in response to numerous postdischarge questions about the availability of community services.

Strategies for Facilitating the Transition

There are some ways to make the transition easier.

The patient is a person with ongoing health care needs that do not end after hospital discharge. Clinicians often view inpatient care as a discrete event, where their chief responsibility is to accomplish the tasks necessary to get the patient out of the acute care setting. "My goal as a resident was to get the patient out of the hospital. Then they were no longer my problem," a physician tells us. Providers need to think not only about treating the medical crisis, but also about promoting healing and wellness. To accomplish this, they must assess factors that may have contributed to the illness or that could contribute to a recurrence. This patient-centered approach requires a long-term perspective that promotes continuity of care.

Continuity of care for patients is frequently lacking when they make the transition from the hospital to the community or alternative care facility. This problem is difficult to address, because no single health care delivery agency is responsible for the follow-up of the recently discharged patient. The hospital's commitment to the patient's well-being ends too often at the moment of discharge, while the primary physician may be unprepared to coordinate the patient's complex home care and psychosocial needs. Hospitals must take the lead in facilitating the transition from the hospital to the community. Posthospital care planning should include a follow-up component to ensure that patients are receiving adequate services and education. In one study, one-third of the patients reported that they needed services postdischarge that they did not receive, and the authors concluded that "the emphasis of discharge planning appears to be more on meeting hospital administrative demands to facilitate speedy discharge than on providing comprehensive care for patients after leaving the hospital" (Wolock, Schlesinger, Dinerman, and Seaton, 1987, p. 71).

It is in the hospital's best interest to promote the well-being of its patients during hospitalization and after discharge, because of the benefits that can be gained in reduced costs, decreased lengths of stay, and increased consumer satisfaction. As one family member told us, "More could be done in the home. . . . Because there is no ancillary care, people have to wait until they're very sick or until they're found somewhere—for example, an old person who is home alone—until they're very, very sick. Then they're in the hospital, and it's a little too late. . . . If a hospital has a supportive facility with pre- and posthospital care, the better they are, and the less hospitalization." In a competitive marketplace, satisfied patients are also the hospital's best advertisement.

This patient-centered perspective is reflected in the nurse case management program at St. Mary's Hospital in Tucson, Arizona. Their nurse case management system was developed to facilitate discharge, provide improved quality of care after hospitalization, decrease readmission rates, and promote cost containment. A nurse case manager coordinates transitional planning with hospitalized patients at high risk for readmission and then coordinates their care in the community. Such nursing services are not reimbursed by third-party payers, although the program's supporters believe it saves the hospital the expense of unreimbursed readmissions (Lamb, 1990).

Follow-up of patients discharged from the hospital may not completely fulfill the goal of continuity of care, but it at least helps to bridge the transition from the hospital to the community. At Wilson Memorial Hospital in Johnson City, New York, primary nurses developed discharge plans, made referrals as necessary, planned education in consultation with their patients, and made home visits to patients recovering from myocardial infarction (Fell, 1979). According to hospital administration, this transition process has changed over time, so that a discharge planning nurse and the patient determine future needs on an individual basis. Home visits to new mothers are also conducted by obstetrical nurses.

Telephone postdischarge interventions may also provide an efficient method of patient follow-up and education. At an experimental program at Wishard Memorial Hospital in Indianapolis, Indiana, nurses called patients after discharge to review unmet needs, discuss medication, and review scheduled appointments. Patients also received informational mailings and appointment reminders. While the intervention group had fewer nonelective readmission days compared to a control group, the results were not statistically significant (Smith, Weinberger, Katz, and Moore, 1988). High-risk patients in the intervention group had significantly higher outpatient costs but lower inpatient costs than those in the control group (Weinberger, Smith, Katz, and Moore, 1988), but these cost savings were not considered enough to justify continuing the intervention beyond the research period.

A similar follow-up program is in place at Newport Hospital in Newport, Rhode Island, in which a nurse telephones rehabilitation patients after hospital discharge to assist with problems and questions regarding home care services, medications, diet, and follow-up. The postdischarge call is made by the same nurse who conducts the preadmission testing and oversees the discharge planning process. At Salem Hospital in Salem, Oregon, volunteers in the "Telecare" program call individuals living at home alone if they have not called the hospital to check in between 9:00 and 11:00 A.M.

Imagine an elderly woman living alone—whose mobility is temporarily limited because of a stroke or a broken hip—coming home from the hospital. How will she feed herself? How will she get to the bathroom? Many patients need direct home care services as part of their postdischarge care and cannot be discharged from the hospital without it. Several hospitals have initiated programs to provide these services for their patients who are at risk for prolonged hospitalization or readmission. Mount Sinai Medical Center in New York offers the Interim Home Care Plan. This program provides intensive home health aide services, which typically involve four to twelve hours of care per day by a trained aide for six to eight weeks. The aide is supervised by a visiting nurse but does not perform skilled nursing care. The program has been judged successful in decreasing the length of stay, promoting continuity of care, and improving the patient's functional status (Schwartz, Blumenfield, and Simon, 1990).

Providing services on a more modest scale, Project Transition at El Camino Hospital in Mountain View, California, helps elderly patients discharged from the hospital to ease the transition from hospital to home. A volunteer visits the patient at home on the day of discharge to run errands, arrange needed services, and coordinate the physician, hospital services, and community and home health agencies (Fleming, 1987). According to the project coordinator, these services have been expanded to include former El Camino Hospital patients who are being discharged from skilled nursing facilities to home. In the future, the support service may be provided to emergency room patients who are not admitted for hospitalization. The mostly volunteer staff helps contain the cost of Project Transition, while this visible community service improves the hospital's image. The most difficult problem facing this program is recruiting enough volunteers.

Rather than providing direct services to patients who live at some distance, the Mayo Clinic in Rochester, Minnesota, has a Transitional Care Unit, which is a converted ward for patients and guests who require limited nursing and support services. This unit was designed primarily for inpatients who need assistance with transition to the home environment, but it is also available for outpatients and elderly or disabled family members. The unit offers hotel services, plus up to two hours of nursing care per day, with an emphasis on education.

Allow enough time for planning. Preparing the patient and family for discharge often starts too late during the hospitalization. Transition planning should not be viewed as something done five minutes before the patient leaves the hospital. Whether it is arranging a nursing home placement or educating the patient on life-style modification, the process should start early. It is easier to deal with problems when they are anticipated in advance. "Early" may be at the time of admission or even before an elective admission.

Efficient planning for posthospital care improves the quality of patient-centered care and helps prevent excessive lengths of stay. It is estimated that 30 percent of hospitalized patients experience delays in discharge (Selker, Beshansky, Pauker, and Kassirer, 1989). The most frequent causes of delays are scheduling of tests (31 percent), unavailability of postdischarge facilities (18 percent), physician decision making (13 percent), and discharge planning (12 percent). In a study of patients with a cerebral vascular accident, congestive heart failure, or hip fracture (Proctor and Morrow-Howell, 1990), 61 percent had at least one complication to discharge planning, according to the social worker interviewed. Common complications were financial impediments, patient confusion, or Medicare/Medicaid coverage restrictions.

Health care providers are not spending enough time discussing postdischarge care. Patients in the Picker/Commonwealth survey were asked how much time during their hospitalization health care providers spent discussing what to do at home. Twenty-two percent of the patients said their physicians spent less than five minutes, and 37 percent said the nurses spent less than five minutes. Disturbingly, patients in fair or poor health more often reported spending less than five minutes with their physician (27 percent) than did those in excellent health (18 percent) (Walker, 1991).

Several hospitals have implemented preadmission screening programs to get a head start on identifying problems with discharge or posthospital care. At Mount Sinai Hospital in New York, a list of patients scheduled for elective surgery is forwarded to the social work department. A volunteer then telephones patients (or their families) who are sixty-five or older or who have specific diagnoses to ask questions such as, "Who will help you when you come home from the hospital?" These calls can both alleviate potential problems and identify patients needing intervention. Patients considered at risk are then referred to a social worker (Simon, 1990).

A pilot program at New England Medical Center's orthopedics and surgical service in Boston confirmed the benefits of a preadmission intervention (Berkman and others, 1988). In this case, elective surgery patients identified as "high risk" by the social service department were telephoned before admission. On follow-up four months after discharge, these patients reported fewer problems with home management and better access to resources than a comparison high-risk group that was screened within the first forty-eight hours in the hospital. Although patients felt that the program had positive benefits, it was discontinued because it was not found to have a significant impact on length of stay.

A similar program is run by nurses at Clinton Memorial Hospital in Wilmington, Ohio. In the preadmission testing program, a nurse is responsible for completing assessment and education for surgical patients prior to admission. Part of her job is to contact the social work department if she anticipates problems related to hospital discharge.

Another approach is to initiate planning for posthospital care early in the admission. For example, patients at Jackson-Madison County General Hospital in Tennessee do not wait to see social workers in the nursing units; they are screened in the admitting office by nurses who identify high-risk cases and refer them immediately to the social service department (Campbell, 1991). At St. Mary Medical Center in Gary, Indiana, social workers identify patients who are "high risk" for discharge problems within forty-eight hours of admission. The social worker assesses psychosocial information and develops a posthospital plan with the patient. The intervention was credited with decreasing lengths of stay by 5.5 days for patients waiting for nursing home placement (Cunningham, 1981).

Early assessment of the patient's needs and concerns should be an integral part of any program to facilitate the transition out of the hospital. While we applaud these interventions for their early identification processes, we emphasize that early assessment should be done for *every* patient, not just those considered to be at "high risk" for excessive lengths of stay or early readmission. The goal of these programs should be to benefit the patient, and the program's success should be measured in terms of its beneficial impact on the patient.

Improve coordination within the hospital and between hospital and community. Patients complain that services are fragmented. Patients and their families are frequently unaware of available resources or are unable to obtain services because they have difficulty negotiating a complex system. Planning and implementing postdischarge care requires contributions from many individuals, both inside and outside of the hospital. Because of the complexity of this process, coordination is essential to ensure that patients receive the needed information and services with a minimum of aggravation.

A multilevel organizational commitment to smooth service delivery must start with senior management. The organizational planning should be interdisciplinary and involve physicians, nurses, and social workers. A multidisciplinary approach to planning for posthospital care helps promote a coordinated effort and fortify a multilevel commitment. Management should ensure that roles are well defined and prevent "turf" issues from interfering with effective implementation. Senior managers must convey the message throughout the organization that *the patient is the focus,* both during hospitalization and after discharge.

Patients should not be "dumped" on community agencies. Planning with communication and coordination between the hospital and outside agencies is essential to the facilitation of the transition out of the hospital. The hospital has a responsibility to ensure that this coordinated effort transpires in a patient-focused manner.

One of the simplest interventions merely requires an addition to the patient chart. "Impediments to Discharge" is a category in the patient chart at Mount Sinai Medical Center in New York. This information is coded, computerized, and updated daily. This encourages a multidisciplinary emphasis on transition planning throughout hospitalization.

The "geriatric evaluation team" is an example of a comprehensive, multidisciplinary program to improve the health, functional status, and social support of elderly patients. This more comprehensive approach illustrates the patient-centered care concept and has been implemented in various hospital settings (Barker and others, 1985; Caradoc-Davies, Dixon, and Campbell, 1989; Rubenstein and others, 1984; Saltz and others, 1988). Although not all of these projects have documented improved patient outcomes, they show potential and are worthy of consideration.

Several hospitals have developed a comprehensive transition planning protocol with a gerontological nurse specialist. At Scott and White Memorial Hospital in Temple, Texas, a gerontological nurse specialist meets with the patient, family, and health care providers to assess resources and support networks available to the patient after discharge. The nurse assists in coordination of services and communication with the patient and family. Once a week, a multidisciplinary team of physicians, physical therapists, social workers, and discharge planners for a specific unit meet to determine posthospitalization needs of the patient. A follow-up visit is made to assess the continuing appropriateness of the discharge plans. The intervention group had a statistically significant shorter average length of stay by two days, as compared to controls. There was no significant difference between the readmission rates among the two groups (Kennedy, Neidlinger, and Scroggins, 1987).

Another comprehensive transition planning protocol implemented by a gerontological nurse specialist at an urban medical center included the following features: (1) comprehensive assessment of the patient's unique needs within twenty-four hours of admission, (2) projection of the patient's postdischarge needs within twenty-four hours of admission, (3) validation of the patient's and caregiver's understanding of the knowledge and skills needs postdischarge, (4) a minimum of two visits during hospitalization by the gerontological nurse specialist for discharge planning, (5) updating the discharge plan twenty-four hours prior to discharge and continued follow-up for two weeks postdischarge, and (6) a minimum of two telephone contacts with the patient during the two weeks after discharge. The experimental group had significantly fewer rehospitalizations, but no significant differences were found in lengths of stay, cost of initial hospitalization, or rates of posthospital infections (Naylor, 1990).

A hospital-based social work consultation service is a potential model to address patient psychosocial problems within the community. Private physicians could consult with the social work department to obtain advice, outreach services, direct services, referral to a community-based program, or follow-up (Blumenfield and Rosenberg, 1988). This model illustrates how hospitals can promote coordination of services and act as a resource to patients and providers in the community.

Summary

Planning for posthospital care requires a systematic, multilevel, interactive process that includes assessment, education, counseling, coordination, and follow-up. Currently, patients report that they are not receiving adequate information or psychosocial support to prepare them for the transition out of the hospital. They want more involvement in the planning process.

Hospital care providers must recognize that patients have ongoing health concerns that do not end on discharge from the hospital. Patient-centered care views the hospitalization as a single "incident" along a continuum of health care.

Planning for posthospital care is a complex, time-consuming process involving multiple providers. Transition planning should begin early during hospitalization, or even before elective admissions. A multilevel commitment to facilitating the transition out of the hospital is needed throughout the organization, starting with top management. This effort must ensure adequate coordination, both within the organization and between the hospital and outside agencies.

Suggestions for Improvement

- Telephone patients scheduled for hospitalization *prior* to admission to identify posthospital needs and concerns.

- Include a "posthospital needs" category on the patient chart to be updated throughout the hospitalization.
- Show patients a videotape about planning for posthospital care, which includes examples of common problems encountered following hospitalization and information on resources to facilitate the transition.
- Increase patient responsibility so that the hospital experience more closely mimics the "real world." For example, encourage patients to administer their own medications or construct their own menus.
- Encourage patients to write down questions they want to ask at their discharge interviews. Do not discharge them until the interviews have been conducted and all questions have been answered.
- Individualize discharge instructions by including a copy of the discharge summary, medication cards, or an audiotape or videotape of the discharge interview.
- Develop a system of nursing and social services to bridge the gap between the hospital and the community. Incorporate transition planning and follow-up with home visits or posthospital consultations. Consider assigning nurse or social work case managers to provide care both in the hospital and in the community.
- Telephone patients after discharge from the hospital to provide education and support and to review unmet needs.
- Offer a telephone information service to answer questions and provide information about community resources.
- Use volunteers or home health aides to facilitate the transition to home.
- Organize multidisciplinary committees to plan and evaluate programs to facilitate the transition out of the hospital. Include patients and family members on the committee.

References

Abramson, J. S. "Enhancing Patient Participation: Clinical Strategies in the Discharge Planning Process." *Social Work in Health Care*, 1990, *14*(4), 53–71.

Anderson, G. F., and Steinberg, E. P. "Hospital Readmissions in the Medicare Population." *New England Journal of Medicine,* 1984, *311*(21), 1349–1353.

Bailey, W. C., and others. "Promoting Self-Management in Adults with Asthma: An Overview of the UAB Program." *Health Education Quarterly,* 1987, *14*(3), 345–355.

Barker, W. H., and others. "Geriatric Consultation Teams in Acute Hospitals: Impact on Back-Up of Elderly Patients." *Journal of American Geriatrics Society,* 1985, *33*(6), 422–428.

Berkman, B., and Abrams, R. D. "Factors Related to Hospital Readmission of Elderly Cardiac Patients." *Social Work,* 1986, *31,* 99–103.

Berkman, B., and others. "Preadmission Screening: An Efficacy Study." *Social Work in Health Care,* 1988, *13*(3), 35–51.

Blumenfield, S., and Rosenberg, G. "Towards a Network of Social Health Services: Redefining Discharge Planning and Expanding the Social Work Domain." *Social Work In Health,* 1988, *13*(4), 31–48.

Campbell, A. W. "Team Works for Continuity." *Picker/Commonwealth Report,* 1991, *1*(1), 9.

Caradoc-Davies, T. H., Dixon, G. S., and Campbell, A. J. "Benefit from Admission to a Geriatric Assessment and Rehabilitation Unit: Discrepancy Between Health Professional and Client Perception of Improvement." *Journal of American Geriatrics Society,* 1989, *37,* 25–28.

Coulton, C. J., Dunkle, R. E., Goode, R. A., and MacIntosh, J. "Discharge Planning and Decision Making." *Health and Social Work,* 1982, 7(4), 253–261.

Cunningham, L. S. "Early Assessment for Discharge Planning." *Quality Review Bulletin,* 1981, 7(10), 11–16.

Dubler, N. N. "Improving the Discharge Planning Process: Distinguishing between Coercion and Choice." *Gerontologist,* 1988, *28,* 76–81.

Fell, P. E. "Home Visits to Evaluate Planning." *American Journal of Nursing,* 1979, *79*(8), 1452–1454.

Fink, A., and others. "Assuring the Quality of Health Care for

Older Persons—An Expert Panel's Priorities." *Journal of American Medical Association,* 1987, *258*(14), 1905-1908.

Fleming, S. "Supporting the Family's Role in Patient Recovery, Rehabilitation." *Promoting Health,* 1987, *8* (Supplement), 1-12.

Jones, E. W., Densen, P. M., and Brown, S. D. "Posthospital Needs of Elderly People at Home: Findings from an Eight-Month Follow-Up Study." *Health Services Research,* 1989, *24*(5), 643-664.

Kennedy, L., Neidlinger, S., and Scroggins, K. "Effective Comprehensive Discharge Planning for Hospitalized Elderly." *Gerontologist,* 1987, *27*(5), 577-580.

Lamb, G. S. "Beyond Discharge: Nurse Case Management for Patients at Risk." Paper presented at Picker/Commonwealth Patient-Centered Care Conference, New Orleans, May 1990.

Lindenberg, R. E., and Coulton, C. "Planning for Posthospital Care: A Follow-Up Study." *Health and Social Work,* 1980, *5*(1), 45-50.

McGinty, M. K., Chase, S. L., and Mercer, M. E. "Pharmacy-Nursing Discharge Counseling Program for Cardiac Patients." *American Journal of Hospital Pharmacy,* 1988, *45,* 1545-1548.

McPhee, S. J., and others. "Influence of a 'Discharge Interview' on Patient Knowledge, Compliance, and Functional Status After Hospitalization." *Medical Care,* 1983, *21*(8), 755-767.

Naylor, M. D. "Comprehensive Discharge Planning for Hospitalized Elderly: A Pilot Study." *Nursing Research,* 1990, *39*(3), 156-161.

Proctor, E. K., and Morrow-Howell, N. "Complications in Discharge Planning with Medicare Patients." *Health and Social Work,* 1990, *15*(1), 45-54.

Rosenbaum, E. E. *The Doctor.* New York: Ballantine Books, 1988.

Rubenstein, L. Z., and others. "Effectiveness of a Geriatric Evaluation Unit—A Randomized Clinical Trial." *New England Journal of Medicine,* 1984, *311*(26), 1664-1670.

Safran, C., and Phillips, R. "Interventions to Prevent Readmission—The Constraints of Cost and Efficacy." *Medical Care,* 1989, *27*(2), 204-211.

Saltz, C. C., and others. "Impact of a Geriatric Consultation Team on Discharge Placement and Repeat Hospitalization." *Gerontologist,* 1988, *28*(3), 344–350.

Schwartz, P. J., Blumenfield, S., and Simon, E. P. "The Interim Home Care Program: An Innovative Discharge Planning Alternative." *Health and Social Work,* 1990, *15*(2), 152–160.

Selker, H. P., Beshansky, J. R., Pauker, S. G., and Kassirer, J. P. "The Epidemiology of Delays in a Teaching Hospital: The Development and Use of a Tool That Detects Unnecessary Hospital Days." *Medical Care,* 1989, *27*(2), 112–129.

Shine, M. S. "Discharge Planning for the Elderly Patient in the Acute Care Setting." *Nursing Clinics of North America,* 1983, *18*(2), 403–410.

Simon, E. P. "Helping Patients in the Hospital Reconnect with Their Lives." Paper presented at Picker/Commonwealth Patient-Centered Care Conference, New Orleans, May 1990.

Smith, D. M., Weinberger, M., Katz, B., and Moore, P. S. "Postdischarge Care and Readmissions." *Medical Care,* 1988, *26*(7), 699–708.

Sumpmann, M. "An Education Center for Patients' High-Tech Learning Needs." *Patient Education and Counseling,* 1989, *13,* 309–323.

Walker, J. D. "What Patients Say About Discharge Planning." *Picker/Commonwealth Report,* 1991, *1*(1), 6.

Weinberger, M., Smith, D. M., Katz, B. P., and Moore, P. "The Cost-Effectiveness of Intensive Postdischarge Care." *Medical Care,* 1988, *26*(11), 1092–1102.

Williams, E. I., and Fitton, F. "Factors Affecting Early Unplanned Readmission of Elderly Patients to Hospital." *British Medical Journal,* 1988, *297*(22), 1039–1043.

Wolock, I., Schlesinger, E., Dinerman, M., and Seaton, R. "The Posthospital Needs and Care of Patients: Implications for Discharge Planning." *Social Work in Health Care,* 1987, *12*(4), 61–76.

PART II

Promoting
a Patient-Centered
Health Care Environment

10

Culture, Leadership, and Service in the Patient-Centered Hospital

Margaret Gerteis
Marc J. Roberts

Whether hospitals know it or not, their reputations for patient-centered care precede them. Patients are as well informed and candid about hospitals known for their kindness and sensitivity as they are about those known for their technical expertise in a particular clinical subspecialty. And patients balance these considerations when they weigh their alternatives (Steiber, 1988). As one focus-group participant, who had undergone the same procedure at two different academic health centers, observed: "If I had to . . . say which hospital would I rather be in? To stay in bed, I'd rather be in [the second hospital]. To do the angioplasty, I'd rather be in [the first]. If they could do the angioplasty and then transfer me over to [the second hospital] again, I would be very, very happy. But that can't be done."

What accounts for the differences that make some hospitals palpably better places, from a patient's point of view, than others?

Our focus so far in this book has been on the individual components of patient-centered care. We have tried to suggest a structured way to think about patients' experiences and the factors that affect the quality of that experience. We have also identified some common problems patients encounter and some of the solutions caregivers have devised to overcome them. Now, we step back and switch lenses, so to speak, to look at the larger environment of the institutions themselves. Our first task is a descriptive one: what does our national survey of hospital patients tell us about the institutional landscape of patient-centered care? With this map in mind, we then examine the characteristics that make hospitals patient centered and their practical implications for managers trying to create more patient-centered institutions.

The Landscape of Patient-Centered Care

Our national survey of hospital patients revealed three striking features of the institutional landscape:

First, the quality of patient-centered hospital care is an institutional characteristic that transcends any particular program or activity. We set out to conduct the Picker/Commonwealth national survey not only to learn more about patients and their experiences, but to find out what it was that good hospitals were doing in the hope that such practices might be replicated elsewhere. We looked for patterns of performance that suggested strength in one or more dimensions of patient-centered care, and we then tried to find innovative programs and practices that accounted for these strong points.

To some extent, our findings confirmed our expectations. The bar graphs in Figure 10.1 offer a profile of the five lowest-performing hospitals we surveyed (in this case, those with the lowest proportion of patients who said they would return to the same hospital, if they had to be hospitalized in the future) and the five highest-performing ones (those with the highest proportion of patients so reporting). Each bar depicts the percentage of patients reporting a problem on certain marker questions within each of the seven dimensions of patient-centered care. The peaks and valleys in each profile reveal, as we suspected, that each hospital has its own internal areas of relative strength and weakness. Yet the more striking feature of these data is that the hospitals tend to fare comparatively better or worse across *all* dimensions of care. Moreover, while the survey hospitals we visited indeed boasted many imaginative programs, some of which are described in earlier chapters, these activities alone were rarely unique or creative enough to explain the differences in overall performance. Even hospitals that did

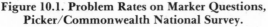

Figure 10.1. Problem Rates on Marker Questions, Picker/Commonwealth National Survey.

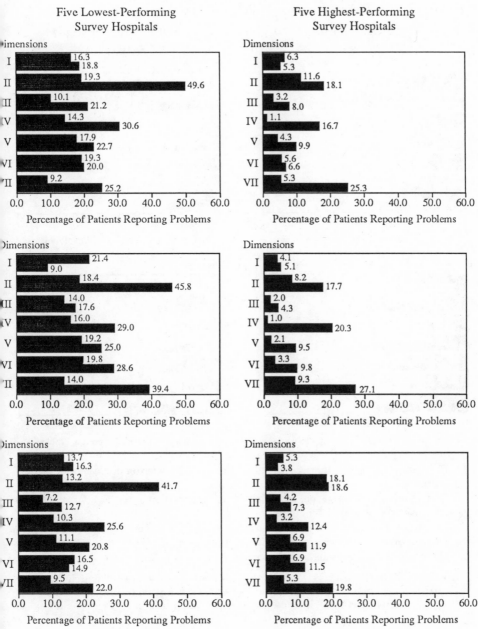

Five Lowest-Performing
Survey Hospitals

Dimensions

I 16.3 / 18.8
II 19.3 / 49.6
III 10.1 / 21.2
IV 14.3 / 30.6
V 17.9 / 22.7
VI 19.3 / 20.0
VII 9.2 / 25.2

Percentage of Patients Reporting Problems

Dimensions

I 21.4 / 9.0
II 18.4 / 45.8
III 14.0 / 17.6
IV 16.0 / 29.0
V 19.2 / 25.0
VI 19.8 / 28.6
VII 14.0 / 39.4

Percentage of Patients Reporting Problems

Dimensions

I 13.7 / 16.3
II 13.2 / 41.7
III 7.2 / 12.7
IV 10.3 / 25.6
V 11.1 / 20.8
VI 16.5 / 14.9
VII 9.5 / 22.0

Percentage of Patients Reporting Problems

Five Highest-Performing
Survey Hospitals

Dimensions

I 6.3 / 5.3
II 11.6 / 18.1
III 3.2 / 8.0
IV 1.1 / 16.7
V 4.3 / 9.9
VI 5.6 / 6.6
VII 5.3 / 25.3

Percentage of Patients Reporting Problems

Dimensions

I 4.1 / 5.1
II 8.2 / 17.7
III 2.0 / 4.3
IV 1.0 / 20.3
V 2.1 / 9.5
VI 3.3 / 9.8
VII 9.3 / 27.1

Percentage of Patients Reporting Problems

Dimensions

I 5.3 / 3.8
II 18.1 / 18.6
III 4.2 / 7.3
IV 3.2 / 12.4
V 6.9 / 11.9
VI 6.9 / 11.5
VII 5.3 / 19.8

Percentage of Patients Reporting Problems

Figure 10.1. Problem Rates on Marker Questions,
Picker/Commonwealth National Survey, Cont'd.

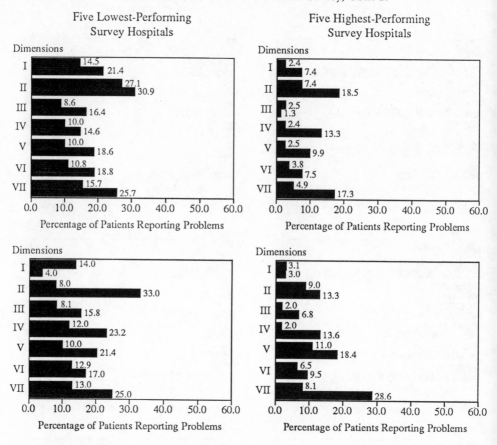

Five Lowest-Performing
Survey Hospitals

Five Highest-Performing
Survey Hospitals

Dimension I = respect for patients' values, preferences, and expressed needs
Dimension II = coordination and integration of care
Dimension III = information, communication, and education
Dimension IV = physical comfort
Dimension V = emotional support and alleviation of fear and anxiety
Dimension VI = involvement of family and friends
Dimension VII = transition and continuity

Note: The Picker/Commonwealth Survey instrument, which was used to generate the information depicted in this figure, contains 58 items querying patients about hospital experiences that might have been problem-

**Figure 10.1. Problem Rates on Marker Questions,
Picker/Commonwealth National Survey, Cont'd.**

atic for them. The following items were selected here, from among those that correlated with patients' decisions about returning to the hospital in the future, to illustrate differences in hospital performance in each dimension:

Dimension I

    Item 1. "Were you involved in the decisions about your care as much as you wanted, or not?"

    Item 2. "Did the doctors sometimes talk in front of you as if you weren't there?"

Dimension II

    Item 1. "Was there one particular doctor in charge of your care in the hospital, or not?"

    Item 2. "Were there times when the nurses were overworked and too busy to take care of you?"

Dimension III

    Item 1. "Consider important questions about your care that you wanted to ask your doctor about. Did you get answers you could understand, or not?"

    Item 2. "Did a doctor or nurse explain the results of the tests in a way you could understand, or not?"

Dimension IV

    Item 1. "When you needed help going to the bathroom, did you get it in time, or not?"

    Item 2. "Could much of your pain have been eliminated by prompt attention by hospital staff, or not?" (asked of patients who reported having pain)

Dimension V

    Item 1. "Did you have a relationship of confidence and trust with the doctor in charge of your treatment at the hospital, or not?"

    Item 2. "Did anyone at the hospital go out of their way to help you or make you feel better, or not?"

Dimension VI

    Item 1. "Was your family given enough information about your hospital care, too much information, or too little information?"

    Item 2. "Was your family or care partner given all the information they needed to help you recover at home, or not?"

Dimension VII

    Item 1. "Did someone in the hospital try and help you with those worries, or not?" (asked of patients who reported having serious worries about problems or difficulties they might have after leaving the hospital)

    Item 2. "Were you told what danger signals about your illness or operation to watch for after you got home, or not?"

not do so well on the survey could often point to similarly creative programs in their own institutions.

A hospital's patient-centeredness is thus much more than the sum of its parts. It is as much (if not more) a function of the hospital's overall culture, mission, and system design and operation as it is the result of particular programs or practices. Promoting patient-centered care therefore requires more than identifying and replicating good practices. We need to understand these more general institutional qualities and how they work.

Second, some environments are more conducive to patient-centered care than others. One of the most obvious features of our hospital survey data is that almost all of the top-performing hospitals—including those profiled in Figure 10.1—are nonteaching hospitals (or hospitals with small teaching programs) located in small, relatively homogeneous communities. This is hardly surprising. It is much easier, after all, to understand patients' preferences and respect their values when everyone, staff and patients alike, shares the same cultural background. It is easier to be sympathetic and supportive when patients, their friends, and their families are likely to be among one's own friends and neighbors. It is easier to coordinate care, communicate effectively, and run an efficient operation when the organization is small, its services limited, and lines of clinical responsibility simple and straightforward. And, of course, it is easier to establish a unanimity of purpose around patient care when there are no competing demands for research, education, jobs, or shelter.

At the other end of the spectrum are the large urban academic health centers that must balance the myriad interests of clinical specialists, medical educators, academic researchers, politicians or government officials, and a community that may be deeply divided by class, race, and ethnicity. Byzantine lines of authority and governance typically connect the administration of the hospital with the medical school, the parent university, and in public institutions, spread out to involve civil service systems, government bureaucracies, and even local legislative processes. Urban public general hospitals may also serve not only as providers of last resort for the neediest, but also as employers of last resort and repositories of patronage. Again, it is not surprising that many of the low-performing survey hospitals are urban academic health centers and that public academic health centers often fared worst of all.

Figure 10.2 graphically depicts the distribution of average "problem rates" among the hospitals we surveyed—that is, the total number of problems reported by patients surveyed from each hospital, divided by the total number of possible problems that could have been reported—grouped by hospital type. Each line represents the total range of problem rates within a particular hospital group, x marks the mean problem rate within that group, and the box delimits the interquartile range within which the hospitals between the 25th and the 75th percentiles in each group fell. Here, the influence of institutional environment is clear: as a group, academic health centers, and especially public academic health centers, experienced the highest problem rates; nonteaching hospitals experienced the lowest problem rates; and other teaching hospitals, as a group, fell in the middle.

We must acknowledge, then, that many of the observable differences among hospitals are the result of external environment as well as institutional culture; that not every aspect of an organization's culture is amenable to change (Schein, 1985); and that managing patient-centered care is, quite simply, objectively more difficult in some environments than in others.

Third—and more important—management is critical to performance, regardless of the environment. From a managerial perspective, the more important feature of the data depicted in Figure 10.2 is that the interquartile range *within* each category is larger than the differences *between* most categories. Clearly, then, factors other than environment are at work in shaping the quality of patient-centered care in these institutions, and these are potentially amenable to managerial intervention.

What Makes Hospitals Patient Centered?

Let us now turn our attention to the characteristics we found to be identified with patient-centered hospitals and consider their implications for managers within different institutional environments.

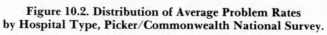

**Figure 10.2. Distribution of Average Problem Rates
by Hospital Type, Picker/Commonwealth National Survey.**

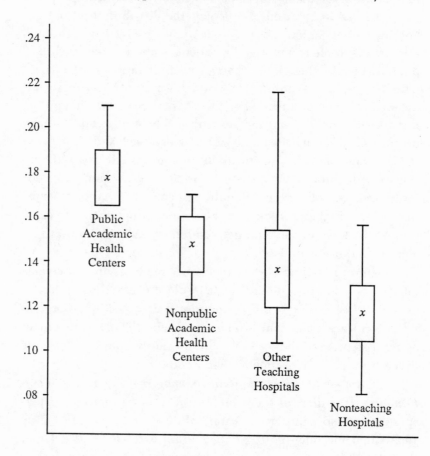

Mission and Culture

The concept of "culture" as an attribute of organizations, as well as of nations and communities, has attracted considerable attention in the management field in recent years. It explains otherwise perplexing and elusive aspects of organizational behavior—the philosophy that shapes relations with employees or outside clients, the unspoken norms that govern behavior, the values that members of the organization seem to share, the "rules of the game," and the climate or "feel" of the place (Schein, 1985). The term is used, variously, to mean any and all of these things. As Schein points out, however, culture in the true sense is deeper and more fundamental. It is the sum total of beliefs and assumptions that operate at an unconscious level among all members of the organization, reinforced by the history and tradition of the institution, the shared experiences of those who work (and have worked) there, and the values, mores, and social structure of the outside community.

Patient-centeredness, in the hospitals we visited, is an expression of organizational culture, in this fundamental sense. Every hospital exists to serve patients. But the successful hospitals we visited exhibited a remarkable unanimity of purpose, extending beyond formal mission statements or official rhetoric. Whether expressed in religious, social, or medical terms, the mission of service in these hospitals is clearly articulated and modeled by top management and permeates every facet of institutional life. It provides the foundation for the sense of professionalism that defines each job in the hospital. Staff at all levels recognize this mission and understand their jobs in terms of it. At Mercy Hospital in Roseburg, Oregon, for example, the chief executive officer at the time of our visit belonged to a religious order and was described by those who worked with her as having the quality of mercy "flowing through her veins." Throughout the hospital, the "spirit of mercy" had an almost palpable quality, incorporated into all strategic planning objectives and self-evaluations. At Jackson-Madison County General Hospital in Jackson, Tennessee, public service to a predominantly Protestant Christian community was similarly defined almost in spiritual terms, in spite of the hospital's secular character. A spokesperson for the Mayo Clinic Foundation in Rochester, Minnesota, describing the clinic's three-part mission of patient care, research, and education, invoked the image of a tricycle, with patient care as the lead "wheel" pulling the other two. Virtually everyone who works at these hospitals, and others like them, understands that service to patients comes first, regardless of competing demands and pressures.

In some small community hospitals, the cultural homogeneity of staff and patients and the relatively small size of the hospital may facilitate this unanimity of purpose and an organizational culture conducive to patient-centered care, although they by no means guarantee it. Larger, more complex institutions, on the other hand, usually serve not one cohesive constituency but many different, and sometimes competing, ones—the most obvious conflicts arising between the demands of clinical teaching or research and those of patient care. Some prestigious academic health centers in fact define their missions first in terms of the advancement of medical science, rather than service to patients. In most larger hospitals, the combination of size, bureaucratic complexity, and specialization also tends to produce fragmented loyalties and professional cultures. A nurse on a pediatric oncology unit, for example, will identify in varying degrees with the unit, the oncology service, the nursing department, and the hospital as a whole, as well as with her professional peers outside the hospital (such as other pediatric oncology nurses) and with the nursing profession. The greater the degree of specialization and bureaucratic complexity, the more numerous and convoluted these nested loyalties and cultures are likely to be (Cooke and Rousseau, 1988; Schein, 1985; Shortell and others, 1991; Coser, 1958, 1962). Many large, complex organizations, in fact, exhibit not one organizational culture, but many different ones, each shaped by different leadership styles, professional values, and behavioral norms (Schein, 1985).

Creating a more patient-centered hospital culture thus presents managers with the double task of promoting patient-centered values in the face of competing missions and defining, nurturing, and sustaining a unified institutional culture in the face of existing—and sometimes stronger—bureaucratic and professional subcultures. Neither task is quickly or easily accomplished. Culture cannot simply be changed to suit our purposes, as Schein (1985) points out, notwithstanding the cavalier statements that appear throughout the popular and academic literature. One recent article about an American Hospital Association hospital "turnaround-of-the-year award," for example, credited the winning institution with creating a "new culture" in a single year (Johnsson and Anderson, 1991)! Whatever else that hospital may have accomplished in one year, it almost certainly did not do that. Culture, by definition, is hard to change. It evolves. It is the living tissue that binds a group or organization together and allows it to survive. Radical culture change may thus be tantamount to destroying the group. And although circumstances may, at times, demand such action, managers must first ask themselves whether it is prudent or practical (Schein, 1985).

A more pragmatic approach is to work within the existing organizational culture to identify a harmony of interests around a defined mission and to build alliances with those in the organization who share those interests. This has been the approach taken by the University of Chicago Hospitals—by tradition, a highly decentralized university-affiliated academic medical center composed of fiercely independent academically based clinical departments, many of them headed by luminaries in the field. The hospital was reconstituted some years ago as a nonprofit medical center administratively independent of the university. The new administration recognized that doing battle with the various departments, in the interest of promoting unity, would be both impractical, given their strength, and strategically unwise, given their importance to the hospital's clinical and academic reputation. Instead, the administration has tried to build on the hospital's and the departments' common interest in attracting and retaining patient referrals in the strongest clinical subspecialties, tapping the strengths of existing professional and departmental subcultures in an effort to create a more patient-centered culture hospitalwide.

Whatever the circumstances, creating a patient-centered culture requires more than a declaration from top administrators. Leaders can set the tone and make their commitment known. But if the mission is to be carried through into practice and forward into the future, it must be a legitimate expression of the organization's values. This, in turn, requires that everyone throughout the organization "buy in" through a process that solicits their genuine involvement. *Everyone* must be involved—not just the yea-sayers—and they must be involved in a way that seriously addresses their interests and concerns. Some members of the organization may eventually "buy out," if their interests are incompatible with the new orientation. Managers may also need, ultimately, to develop strategies to deal head on with the most stubborn pockets of resistance. But defining a patient-centered mission and building the organizational culture that can sustain that mission requires a continuing effort over time. Those whose career paths require quick successes are bound to be frustrated; they may be able to create a flashy stir, but they are unlikely to leave behind an organization with the capacity to carry through its mission.

Human Resources

A hospital's ability to create and sustain a culture conducive to patient-centered care also depends on its ability to attract, retain, and motivate the "right" people and to socialize them into the institutional culture. When we asked managers of high-performing hospitals what they owed their success to, time and again they told us about the pervasive "work ethic," which they often attributed to community values outside the hospital—a "Scandinavian work ethic" in the northern-tier states; a "Protestant work ethic" in the South; "small-town American values" in the Midwest; and, variously, the "pioneer spirit," the farming tradition, or middle-class values. While the denizens of small-town middle America may identify with these Calvinist virtues, managers of inner-city hospitals in large urban melting pots are more likely to notice the deep class divisions, ethnic rivalries, political wheeling and dealing, and chronic social problems that mitigate against any such "work ethic" in their own environments. As one urban hospital executive wrote us after visiting a small-town hospital that performed particularly well on our survey, "Here, there are no AIDS patients, no drug-addicted newborns, . . . no rival gang members working the after-school shift in dietary. . . ." Nor, in all likelihood, were there jobs filled by patronage or "make-work" programs for disadvantaged youth.

Still, the differences in the qualities of work forces are not simply attributable to social environment. The successful hospitals we encountered, whatever their location, clearly invested time and energy recruiting and screening new job applicants. For example, middle and upper managers at Trinity Hospital in Minot, North Dakota, told us that they would rather leave a job vacant than fill it with the wrong person, even though they acknowledged that labor shortages in some areas at times made this a difficult rule to follow. When the Mayo Clinic set up satellite sites in Jacksonville, Florida, and Scottsdale, Arizona, its transplanted managers similarly spent months recruiting and screening staff who could understand and embrace the Mayo philosophy of patient care. Managers may object that local shortages of skilled labor, financial constraints that limit their ability to offer competitive wages and salaries, or legal and social prohibitions against discriminatory hiring practices would preclude selective hiring of this sort in their own milieus. Selective hiring is, by definition, discriminating. But properly done, it allows managers to reassess the skill mixes and staffing ratios they need and helps them avoid the cultural stereotypes or superficial judgments in hiring that lead to discrimination in the negative sense (Schlesinger and Heskett, 1991). It requires them, first, to analyze the nature and purpose of the work to be done and the qualities needed to do it well, and to define appropriate screening criteria based on this assessment. In many cases, formal training and experience may be less relevant to potential performance than an earnest desire to help sick people and a willingness to learn. Many employers now use "value-based interviewing" techniques to help gauge qualities such as compassion, openness to new ways of doing things, or the ability to work as part of a team.

Investing in human resources entails a genuine respect for the work of professional and nonprofessional staff alike. This means far more than heaping praise on employees at annual picnics or ceremonial dinners or launching "smile" campaigns to improve their "attitude" (Deming, 1986; Albrecht and Zemke, 1985). It requires, first of all, a commitment to training and education that gives workers both the skills they need to do their job well and the opportunity to develop personally on the job (Deming, 1986). Schlesinger and Heskett (1991) have cited the example of one food service company that brought in medical professionals to teach entry-level employees about disease transmission. The program was designed not only to teach new workers the basics of food handling and hygiene, but to treat them as professionals and to send the message that management took them and their work seriously. As important, it created an educational opportunity that helped them understand their work in a larger context. Cultivating the sort of work culture that we found conducive to patient-centered care entails an ongoing commitment to the workers who deliver the services. At all of the high-performing hospitals we visited, employees spoke of their hospital's reputation as a "good place to work." Staff at one small public hospital in Ohio told us that theirs were the "best jobs in the county"—an implied comparison that included not only other county jobs, but also those in a thriving local private industry. At the Mayo Clinic, staff at all levels, who have been carefully recruited, trained, and acculturated into the clinic community, can expect to stay for life—and many of them do. Their loyalty is secured, in part, through programs of tuition assistance, for both them and their families; educational courses to enhance their job skills; and support services for their families.

For good or ill, culture endures through processes that are largely self-perpetuating. Workers are attracted to those institutions whose values, working styles, and cultural attributes are consistent with their own.

The Front Lines

The test of a hospital's patient-centeredness is the delivery of service at the "front lines" of patient care. This, in turn, suggests two strategies for managers who want to create more patient-centered institutions. First, as we have argued throughout this book, managers must ask patients to evaluate service performance. And second, managers must understand that those who deliver the service, in every dimension of care, are the ones who will ultimately determine the quality of the performance. To illustrate this point, consultants in the field of quality management often turn the usual hierarchical model of organizational structure upside down. Patients are at the top of this inverted pyramid, followed by the product or service delivery workers at the organization's front ranks, who are in turn "supported" by progressively narrower ranks of line supervisors, middle managers, senior managers, and (finally) the chief executive (Leebov and Scott, 1990).

Yet the message that front-line service is critical suggests a personnel strategy far different from that ordinarily followed by service organizations, including hospitals. Why is this so often such a difficult concept to put into practice? These days, a great deal of the blame is assigned to financial constraints that force hospitals everywhere to focus on the bottom line. In hospitals, as in other labor-intensive service industries, the obvious place to cut is in labor costs, and this is routinely accomplished in several ways: by laying off workers (especially those with least rank or seniority), or allowing their ranks to diminish through attrition; by switching from full-time to part-time staff, to save the costs of full-time benefits; by counting on short tenures and high rates of turnover, to keep wage levels down (Schlesinger and Heskett, 1991; Bane and Ellwood, 1991). Yet these short-term cost-cutting measures will also likely lead to a decline in patient-centered quality and a loss of patients and revenues. The experiences of other service industries are telling in this respect. At Sears, the shift from a 70 percent full-time to a 70 percent part-time sales force correlated directly with a sharp drop in customer satisfaction, because the part-timers were less knowledgeable and therefore less able to handle customers' requests or complaints. Managers at Merck & Company also found the total cost of job turnover—taking into account the disruption of work relationships and the transactional costs of hiring and training new workers—to be about 150 percent of an employee's annual salary (Schlesinger and Heskett, 1991).

The tendency to cut costs at the front lines of service, however, reflects a much more profound problem in the industry than short-term financial constraints. Theodore Levitt (1986) has pointed out that there has been a remarkable lack of creativity in the industrial organization of service, generally, because of the traditional, class-bound, and deep-rooted tendency to equate "service" with one-on-one personal attendance and servility. The result has been both to misconstrue the nature of the work and to undervalue it. Nonprofessional service workers (disproportionately female and minority) occupy a low social status, are paid low wages, and tend to be regarded as eminently replaceable, even interchangeable (Bane and Ellwood, 1991).

The front-line service that matters most from the patient's perspective, apart from clinical treatment, and that most strongly influences their evaluation of a hospital's performance is personal care at the bedside. Data from our national survey suggest that while patients may ultimately forgive hospitals that fail to keep them informed about daily routines or prepare them adequately for discharge, they are less likely to forgive a hospital's failure to meet such basic needs as answering the call button or helping them bathe or go to the bathroom. Patients who reported problems in these areas were about four times more likely to say they would not return to that hospital in the future and nearly nine times more likely not to recommend it to friends or families than those who did not experience such difficulties.

Yet responsibility for the nonclinical aspects of bedside care is often diffuse. By tradition, it has been the domain of nursing, a profession ambivalently poised at the intersection of the clinical and the personal caring aspects of medicine. As nurses have taken on a more autonomous role in clinical care, many of the routine caring functions have been left to others: licensed practical nurses, aides, housekeepers, dietary staff. Although the question has yet to be put to a formal test, our informal observations in the field suggest that there is no optimal mix of players that will maximize the quality of patient-centered care at the bedside. One high-performing hospital we visited followed a primary nursing model of patient care, relying on nurses trained at the baccalaureate and master's level. But hospitals elsewhere that also performed well in the eyes of their patients relied, variously, on two-year nursing graduates, aides trained in-house, even unpaid volunteers, depending in part on their financial resources and the characteristics of the local labor market. What they all shared was a recognition of the primary importance of personal patient care, however it is organized, and a commitment to recruitment, training, and retention of staff to deliver that care. For managers, the task is not only to recognize and support the work of the front lines, but to determine the appropriate combination of players and to coordinate their work effectively, given the constraints of bureaucratic reporting structures, institutional finances, and professional prerogatives.

In hospitals, the issue is complicated by the fact that physicians are the traditionally recognized and legally sanctioned front-line caregivers, notwithstanding the profusion of institutionally based clinical specialties, clinical support services, nursing, and ancillary services now integral to patient care (Harris, 1977). And patients, for the most part, still look to their physicians to be "in charge." When quality management expert W. Edwards Deming witnessed errors and inefficiencies on the part of the nursing staff during his hospitalization, he, like most patients, complained to his doctor (recounted in a memo, 1987). Yet the unique relationship of physicians to hospitals has long intrigued sociologists, organizational theorists, and others interested in the institutional life of American medicine (Freidson, 1970; Coser, 1962; Goss, 1963; Begun, 1985; Harris, 1977; Pauly and Redisch, 1973). Attending physicians rarely have any formal authority over hospital staff, and hospital managers often complain that they have little authority over physicians.

Ironically, however, it is often community-based physicians—those who have the loosest institutional ties—who are most sensitive to hospital patients' subjective needs and experiences, precisely because the competitive pressures of community practice require them to develop such sensitivities. Staff physicians in academic medical centers may be formally employed by the institutions they serve, but they adhere to the cultural norms and respond to the incentive systems of academic medicine, not patient-centered clinical care. In this subculture, house officers are the front-line workers, who respond to the standards of performance set by the chief of the clinical department. One staff physician from an academic medical center participating in our physicians' focus group described the incentives in his own department in the following terms: "There are no rewards, no raises, for paying attention to these issues [patient-centered care] in the system we work with. If anything, the system encourages you to cut corners on this. I mean, patients are not asked systematically what they think of us. On the other hand, medical students are asked at the end of every rotation [about] the person who taught them. If we do well [in teaching], it's noticed, and if we do poorly, certainly attention is paid to that. Similarly, in our research, people count the number of articles we wrote, and they notice the guy who didn't write anything last year.'' Improving the quality of front-line care in these settings thus entails changing the system of incentives.

Systems Management

The ultimate test of a hospital's performance is what its patients experience. A hospital's mission and culture establish its direction; its human resources provide the steam that keeps it going. The third critical ingredient of its performance are the systems, the engineering mechanics, that make it work. No amount of goodwill, motivation, and hard work can make up for systems that do not work (Crosby, 1979; Deming, 1986; Imai, 1986; Carlzon, 1987; Garvin, 1988; Gitlow and Gitlow, 1987; Ishikawa, 1985; Juran, 1964). And yet hospitals that pride themselves, deservingly, on their mission and humanity may pay little attention to the mechanics of their operation, precisely because such a focus seems too mechanistic. One such hospital we visited, held in high esteem for the patient-centered quality of its care and for its enlightened personnel policies, nonetheless exhibited some striking operational failures. Patients and visitors confront a hodgepodge of interconnected buildings and corridors, with very little in the way of directional aids. Patients complain that hospital bills are unfathomable, and yet staff of the collections office, to whom they are directed with their questions, know nothing about how the bills are prepared. Nurses are encouraged and empowered to take responsibility for all aspects of patient care, and yet there is no systematic, informed approach to patient education.

The way to test a hospital's effectiveness in delivering patient-centered care is to ask patients what they experience. Many hospitals now conduct patient satisfaction or opinion surveys as part of their marketing or strategic planning efforts. However, patient-generated data can be an especially useful management tool, providing independent feedback on existing operations, if they extend beyond global ratings of satisfaction or dissatisfaction and provide, instead, explicit feedback about concrete aspects of patients' experience (Cleary and others, 1991; Cleary, Edgman-Levitan, McMullen, and Delbanco, 1992). Different types of feedback may be useful in different types of situations. Focus groups, for example, provide qualitative, open-ended, first-person accounts that can be used to identify problems or test patients' responses to planned initiatives. Videotapes of focus groups are especially persuasive with hospital staff. Paper-and-pencil questionnaires can be used to evaluate units or services against established performance criteria, as the University of Chicago has done in its emergency room (Fullam, 1991), or to survey a large sample of patients across all services on discharge. Telephone interviews conducted shortly after discharge, although more expensive to administer, can improve response rates among large patient samples, provide more detailed information, and overcome problems relating to literacy or bias. The statistically significant quantitative data that well-designed and controlled patient surveys can generate are especially compelling to academic physicians. Feedback from patients not only helps managers identify problems that might otherwise go unnoticed— for example, the problems with directions, billing, and education noted above—but it can also help overcome the professional resistance that comes from investment in established ways of doing things.

Patient-centered systems management also requires the involvement of physicians, both because doctors, too, are important "customers" of the hospital and because, as the traditional primary caregivers, they bear the brunt of responsibility for front-line patient care. And yet even the top-performing hospitals we visited were not very successful at involving physicians in internal administrative operations, decision making, or strategic planning. Most managers told us, for instance, that doctors had not taken part in service quality efforts, although, in some cases, programs had been specifically designed for them. Others were reluctant to give physicians critical feedback from quality assessments, for fear of alienating them. And in some instances, a hospital's failure to involve physicians in planning or decision making led to serious rifts with the attending staff. Time and time again, we heard the common complaint, even from otherwise successful hospitals, that "we haven't been able to get the doctors involved." Unless the locus of provider responsibility shifts markedly away from physicians, in both the public's and the profession's eyes, however, the effectiveness of any efforts to improve the systems for delivering patient-centered services will be limited if physicians do not play a central integrative role (Begun, 1985; Koeck and Levitt, 1990; Charns, 1976). Yet in many respects, the tendency over the past several years has been in precisely the opposite direction. Physicians, leery of cost containment and administrative interference in their practice decisions, have often resisted hospitals' efforts to review and assess quality based on standardized protocols. For their part, too, hospital administrators have been frustrated by physicians' professional autonomy. In response, they have often tried to tighten administrative control over hospital operations, as well as over the physician privileging process (Morlock, Alexander, and Hunter, 1985; Slomski, 1991). Some observers of the health care scene, however, see evidence of a rapprochement between doctors and hospital managers. The systems approach characteristic of total quality management has already begun to shift attention and the burden of responsibility for quality away from individual physician performance, for purposes both of accreditation and professional credentialing (Koska, 1991b; "TQM Likely to Change Focus . . .," 1991). At the same time, more physicians now express an interest in pursuing careers in health care management, in part out of frustration with the tightening constraints on private clinical practice (Koska, 1991a). These trends, too, if they continue, are salutary to the future of patient-centered care.

Middle Management

While senior managers can institute recruitment and selective hiring practices to help find the right people for the job, middle managers and line supervisors are the ones who most directly influence what actually gets done. If workers in the most patient-centered hospitals display a strong work ethic, it is at least in part because their supervisors set high standards of performance and reward those who meet them. At the same time, middle managers who stick to the conventional way of doing things can (and often do) effectively block organizational change, regardless of top management's determination to create a more patient-centered culture (Leebov and Scott, 1990). The head of quality improvement at one large academic health center we visited echoed a familiar sentiment when she described the middle managers in her hospital as falling into three groups of roughly equal size: those who had been explicitly trained for their jobs; those who had been deservedly promoted; and those who had been promoted through the "Peter Principle," until they had reached their level of incompetence. This last group, she said, formed the biggest bloc of resistance to change. Most of them had been at the hospital a long time, and they expected to be there long after the current team of top managers had moved on. But the crux of the oft-cited "problem" of middle management, we would argue, is not so much that their ranks are riddled with incompetents or "deadwood"; it is rather that this group most directly embodies and perpetuates the existing culture. Middle managers have often come up through the ranks, rewarded through promotion for behavior consistent with the existing system of values, the accepted rules of the game. They therefore have both a material and an ethical stake in the existing culture, and they set standards of performance for those they supervise that are consistent with those values.

Middle managers are thus key to the creation of a more patient-centered hospital culture and to the design of effective systems of service delivery. Because they often see them as more of a hindrance than a help to their reform efforts, however, senior managers may be tempted to rely on their own team of newcomers from the outside and to avoid the old guard. But unless middle managers actively buy into the new organizational mission and culture, the actual delivery of front-line patient care will not change. Workers will continue to be rewarded for performing discrete tasks according to established criteria, rather than for delivering patient-centered care. Moreover, middle managers who have come up through the ranks are most familiar with existing operating systems, their strengths, and their failures. If they accept and understand the validity of the patient's perspective, they can therefore be a valuable resource in creating more effective systems of service delivery. Leebov and Scott (1990) discuss at some length the shifting roles of middle managers in changing health care organizations and strategies for converting them from "tradition and safety" to "experimentation and risk." The very qualities that marked some as "mavericks" or "troublemakers" in the past, they point out, may identify those most likely to be valuable allies to reform-minded administrators, because the mavericks have already demonstrated their disgruntlement with standard operating procedures.

Service chiefs in teaching hospitals make up one particularly strong, and traditionally independent, group of middle managers who are especially critical to the quality of patient-centered care. In many hospitals, the departments they administer function as mini-empires, with their own traditions and cultures and with only the loosest sort of ties to the administration of the hospital as a whole. One staff physician from a moderate-sized teaching hospital described the workings of his own department thus:

> The [hospital] administrator's at the top of the system that I'm, in a sense, not even part of. He's the head of the hospital and employs all the hospital workers, but he doesn't employ [doctors]—there's a pretty circuitous route between him and the docs. The medical staff and the house officers relate to the hierarchy within their departments, and that is only in some attenuated way related to the hospital administration. The administration is involved in decisions about who the chief of the department is going to be, but other than that they don't have that much to do with the reward system within a given department. That's established by the department's own rules—even more than the rules, the sort of ethos of the department. The hospital administration doesn't have a great deal of influence on how house officers or staff physicians behave.

Although service chiefs' medical school affiliations and their traditions of professional autonomy make them decidedly a special case, hospital managers must develop strategies for dealing with them, just as they must deal with all middle managers in their ranks, if they hope to succeed in changing the institutional culture.

Conceptually, at least, the problems and the strategies for dealing with them are not dissimilar. The new administration of the University of Chicago, for example, began by allying with the mavericks among the service chiefs—those who were dissatisfied with the existing systems of patient care in the hospital and who had already begun to create more patient-centered cultures in their own departments. Administrators at Jackson-Madison Hospital in Jackson, Tennessee, launched a hospitalwide guest relations program by offering it first to the staff of admitting physicians' private offices. Seeing its benefits firsthand, the doctors in turn supported the hospital's effort, which they might otherwise have dismissed as frivolous. Yet another large academic health center, after failing to convince several particularly obstinate chiefs of service that their medical staff's insensitivity to patients was costing the hospital referrals, began to actively court community-based physicians in those specialties by offering them office space and other amenities.

Environment, Leadership, and Change

We opened this chapter by remarking that some climates are more conducive to patient-centered care than others. But lest we too hastily sing the praises of small community hospitals or curse the task of promoting patient-centered care in urban academic health centers, we must remind ourselves that the hospital environment is radically changing. The future quality and viability of hospitals everywhere, whatever their circumstances, will depend as much or more on their ability to manage and adapt to change as on their past performance or the beneficence of their environment.

The Changing Environment

The forces that once fostered harmony, unity, and simplicity in smaller community hospitals are rapidly eroding. Population shifts and changes in local economies are bringing cultural and economic diversity even to once-insular communities. Roseburg, Oregon, traditionally a town of blue-collar working families, is now attracting relatively well-off retirees from California and points east. Lafayette, Indiana, is now the site of a Toyota assembly plant and home to the families of Japanese-born managers. Virtually all of the small community hospitals we visited spoke, too, of the local scarcity of physicians, nurses, and skilled ancillary workers and of the resulting need to recruit "outsiders" to fill vacancies. Minot, North Dakota, now boasts a Chinese restaurant, owned by the family of one such physician recruited to the area. To the extent that internal harmony in small community hospitals depended, in the past, on the cultural homogeneity of the community, times are changing (Wagner, 1991).

No less than other hospitals in the country, community hospitals have also felt the financial and competitive pressures brought on by changing reimbursement policies and reduced utilization. Hospitals that were flush until a few years ago now worry about their "bottom line" and keep a close watch on physicians' practice patterns. As elsewhere, such pressures have strained relations with attending physicians unaccustomed to such scrutiny. Intensified competition is also bringing an abrupt end to the "gentlemen's agreement" that once partitioned local markets. Even hospitals that used to be the only ball game in town now worry about losing patients to academic health centers twenty, fifty, or a hundred miles away. In response, small hospitals are prompted to add specialty services in an effort to stay in the game, and adding services adds to their administrative complexity as well.

The changing financial and regulatory environment has also altered the corporate structure of community hospitals, bringing growing numbers into multi-institutional hospital systems. Although the particulars of such arrangements vary enormously from one system to another, they have undoubtedly brought the benefits of central planning and centralized services to otherwise isolated, and vulnerable, community hospitals. However, in so doing, they have also shifted the locus of authority over institutional decisions and altered traditional relations between hospital administrators, boards of trustees, and medical staffs. One study found that administrators were held more accountable for hospital operations and that medical staff were less involved in operational decisions in hospitals participating in multi-institutional arrangements, compared with their independent counterparts (Morlock, Alexander, and Hunter, 1985). In this respect too, then, life is no longer so simple for community hospitals, nor are relationships of power and authority so direct as they once were.

Ironically, the same forces that are complicating the environments of small community hospitals may be helping to create climates *more* favorable to patient-centered care in large urban academic health centers. Long before community hospitals felt the pinch, third-party cost containment efforts brought financial turmoil to many of these institutions, and the pressure has often prompted a reexamination of administrative structures and governing relationships. Whether the impetus came from governing bodies no longer willing to bear financial responsibility for the troubled hospitals, or from hospital managers seeking more control over their institutions, the trend toward institutional independence and more simplified lines of authority among academic health centers appears well established (Pallarito, 1990). The University of Chicago Hospitals, for example, severed its administrative ties with the university in 1986 and now operates as an independent, nonprofit hospital. The Regional Medical Center of Memphis, formerly a county-operated public general hospital, also serves now as a "private nonprofit hospital with a public mission," governed by the Shelby County Health Care Corporation board of directors. Similar changes have taken place at other university-affiliated and public general hospitals, moving them toward more simplified administrative structures and management.

The move toward independence has also introduced a sensitivity to the market that was far less apparent when the cushion of university or public financial support was available. As a result, urban academic health centers have begun, of necessity, to view their patients more as customers than as "teaching material" or public wards. The growing interest among academic health centers in patient satisfaction, guest relations, and service excellence programs is testimony to their changing posture in this regard. In other respects, too, the peculiar problems of older urban general hospitals can create opportunities for change. The badly deteriorating physical environment of many older inner-city hospitals, for instance, has prompted a significant investment in new building, and this in turn may provide the occasion and the opportunity for experimental new designs in service delivery. For example, at the Medical

College of Virginia Hospital in Richmond, an experimental 100-bed "minihospital" has been designed as part of a new medical/surgical building, where many hospital services are decentralized and front-line patient care completely reorganized. Even rapid turn-over in top management—a telling characteristic of "troubled" in-stitutions everywhere—can create openings for new leadership and new ideas.

Leadership and Change

The administrator of one small community hospital we visited no doubt echoed the sentiments of many of his colleagues at similar institutions when he told us that he was less concerned about mak-ing his hospital more patient centered—since it already was that way—than about competing on technical grounds with larger nearby teaching hospitals. But the message we would deliver here to community hospitals is that their traditional strength in the hu-mane, nontechnical aspects of care may not be as secure as they think. *The challenge community hospitals face is to maintain and build on their strength in patient-centered care while they adapt to a rapidly changing social and economic environment.*

The experience of Jackson-Madison County General Hospi-tal in Tennessee exemplifies some of the difficulties encountered by small community hospitals when they expand and diversify in re-sponse to increased competition. Until about a decade ago, Jackson-Madison had been a small community hospital serving a homo-geneous, mostly rural area of Tennessee. Then the hospital built a new physical plant, expanded to 600 beds, and began to add a va-riety of specialized services. Staff who lived through the transition described a loss of the cohesive "family" feeling that had once char-acterized the hospital culture and an increasing sense of distance between staff and the now stronger and more centralized adminis-tration. They also saw a growing dissonance between the hospital's new "high-tech" character as a large, modern regional medical cen-ter and the community's traditional expectations of a small-town hospital.

In an effort to restore some of the lost feeling of smallness, the new administration at Jackson-Madison has adopted a two-pronged approach, aimed first at employees and next at patients. Staff at all levels are invited to weekly "grassroots" sessions with the chief executive officer and other senior managers, where they are encouraged to air grievances, ask questions, or comment on any aspect of hospital operations or working life. The administration, in turn, promises to answer every question raised. Creating the occasion for communal discussion, however, is no guarantee that it will take place. Employees in this case, for example, reportedly were slow to speak up, until the format was changed to solicit anonymous, written questions and comments in advance. But through its persistence, the administration has conveyed the seriousness of its intention to change the working culture of the hospital in a way that values staff, their participation, and their feedback. The second prong of this conscious culture shift will address patients' needs and expectations of the hospital.

As smaller community hospitals gear up to invest in new technology and specialized medical services, the same competitive challenges are forcing their technologically sophisticated urban academic neighbors to pay more attention to the human side of the care they deliver. For them, tradition is a hindrance in this respect, not a source of strength. *The challenge academic health centers face is to seize opportunities to create more humane, patient-centered institutions within the constraints of their history, environment, and culture.*

Something of the magnitude of the task in difficult environments is suggested by the recent efforts of the Regional Medical Center of Memphis, Tennessee. In a city sharply divided along class and race lines, the "Med" has suffered most of the ills afflicting urban public general hospitals. It has been a dumping ground for the (mostly black) sick poor, relying entirely on its teaching affiliation with the University of Tennessee Medical School for its (mostly white) medical staffing. To many in public life, the hospital has traditionally been regarded as a publicly subsidized employer of last resort for the city's otherwise unemployable unskilled or marginally trained workers, and the Med's work force has been generally held in poor repute by the city's medical community. The work culture of the hospital was one thus characterized by strong hostilities among administration, medical staff, and the nonmedical work force; low job expectations and low job performance; and poor morale. Over the past several years, the Med's administration has tried to revamp the hospital's reputation and public image, without abandoning its mission of public service either as a medical care provider or as an employer. As it demands and enforces new standards of performance on the job, the Med also recognizes an obligation to assess, teach, and enhance workers' basic job skills. To the extent that it succeeds, it will serve the public function not only of providing employment, but of making marginal members of the labor force more employable. At the same time, the new administration is trying to heighten workers' sense of identity and loyalty to the institution through programs of support, including emergency financial assistance and basic literacy programs. While the Med clearly has a long way to go to solve its problems, the payoff of its new investment in human resources is reportedly visible in improved recruitment, morale, and job performance.

Hospitals vary enormously in their capacity to confront a changing environment. In many favored institutions, the absence of competition or challenge has bred an unwarranted complacency. One community hospital we visited, long the only one in a market area of about 150,000, has remained remarkably unruffled by the aggressive marketing campaigns—complete with television promotions and mass mailings—conducted by several big teaching hospitals within an hour's drive. When we asked how they planned to counter such incursions, the hospital's managers spoke confidently of the "loyalty" of the community and calmly pledged to "continue doing what we've always done." The only response thus far to a declining census and shifting patterns of utilization has been an attempt to increase collections and raise awareness about hospital costs.

By way of contrast, another community hospital in very similar circumstances has been anything *but* complacent about the competing attractions of renowned academic health centers in cities even farther away. "The people in this town tend not to think much about this hospital—*until they come here*," a hospital spokesperson told us. Managers there know they have to prove their worth to the local community. To do so, they have, among other things, enlisted the support of the medical staff to develop quality data and quality improvement feedback mechanisms; designated nursing and social work staff to follow discharged patients in the community; recruited a new chief of anesthesia, who established a hospitalwide pain management program; and set up a comprehensive financial counseling program within the admissions office. Instead of relying on community loyalty or entering a contest with the larger teaching hospitals that it would inevitably lose, this institution has thus built on its strengths as a community hospital to enhance the patient-centered quality of its care.

However favorable or unfavorable its circumstances, then, a hospital's *management* makes a difference in its capacity to face the future, and the quality of its leaders makes a difference. Competent, cautious top managers who can keep things "running smoothly" may be good enough in ordinary times, but extraordinary times—changing and stressful environments—require leadership of a different caliber. They require managers who are as attuned to the world outside the hospital as they are to its internal operations; who understand the larger systems in which the hospital operates; and who can anticipate, for example, changes in the regulatory environment or the demographics of the market or the labor pool, recognize their significance, and develop proactive strategies for dealing with them (Senge, 1990; Johnson, 1991; Marszalek-Gaucher and Coffey, 1990).

Extraordinary times also require leaders who can evoke a transforming vision for the institution and mobilize the internal resources to carry that vision through—who can overcome what Bennis (1989) has described as the "unconscious conspiracy" of an organization to maintain the status quo. And above all, hospitals need people in charge who care enough about the institution to make the commitment of time and energy needed to lead it.

Summary

"Patient-centeredness" in a hospital is more than the sum of good practices or innovative programs. It is, rather, a fundamental feature of institutional culture. Creating and sustaining such a culture requires unity of purpose throughout the organization behind a mission of service and patient care; an ability to attract and retain a work force at all levels whose values are consistent with this mission; a recognition of the importance of front-line service, especially basic bedside care, and of the human resources that provide this service; continuous improvement of the systems of delivery; and a recognition of the critical role middle managers play in setting standards of care and improving delivery systems.

Undeniably, some environments are more conducive to a patient-centered culture than others. Historically, the small size, limited missions, and cultural homogeneity characteristic of small community hospitals have made it easier for them to unite around a consistent set of values and a commitment to patient service. Large urban academic health centers, at the other extreme, have multiple missions, answer to many masters, and serve a large, disparate, and sometimes divided community; these characteristics often make it difficult to build a unified institutional culture. There is, therefore, no "boilerplate" for promoting patient-centered care. Any strategy, to be effective, must take into account the constraints of the existing environment and culture.

And yet the environment is rapidly changing. The advantages that once favored small community hospitals are disappearing, as they lose their insularity and compete with the larger teaching hospitals of the city. The same competitive challenges now force big teaching hospitals to pay more attention than they have in the past to the humane aspects of care. Hospitals cannot afford to rest on their laurels, to do business as usual. The times require visionary leaders with the commitment and tenacity to define and sustain a new mission of high-quality, patient-centered care.

References

Albrecht, K., and Zemke, R. *Service America! Doing Business in the New Economy.* Homewood, Ill.: Dow Jones–Irwin, 1985.

Bane, M. J., and Ellwood, D. T. "Is American Business Working for the Poor?" *Harvard Business Review,* 1991, *69,* 58–66.

Begun, J. W. "Managing With Professionals in a Changing Health Care Environment." *Medical Care Review,* 1985, *42,* 3–10.

Bennis, W. *Why Leaders Can't Lead: The Unconscious Conspiracy Continues.* San Francisco: Jossey-Bass, 1989.

Carlzon, J. *Moments of Truth*. New York: Ballinger, 1987.

Charns, M. P. "Breaking the Tradition Barrier: Managing Integration in Health Care Facilities." *Health Care Management Review*, 1976, *1*, 55–67.

Cleary, P. D., Edgman-Levitan, S., McMullen, W., and Delbanco, T. L. "The Relationship Between Reported Problems and Patient Summary Evaluations of Hospital Care." *Quality Review Bulletin*, 1992, *18*(2), 53–59.

Cleary, P. D., and others. "Patients Evaluate Their Hospital Care: A National Survey." *Health Affairs*, 1991, *10*, 254–267.

Cooke, R. A., and Rousseau, D. M. "Behavioral Norms and Expectations: A Quantitative Approach to the Assessment of Organizational Culture." *Group and Organization Studies*, 1988, *13*, 245–273.

Coser, R. L. "Authority and Decision Making in a Hospital: A Comparative Analysis." *American Sociological Review*, 1958, *23*, 56–63.

Coser, R. L. *Life in the Ward*. East Lansing: Michigan State University Press, 1962.

Crosby, P. B. *Quality Is Free: The Art of Making Quality Certain*. New York: New American Library, 1979.

Deming, W. E. *Out of the Crisis*. Cambridge: Center for Advanced Engineering Study, Massachusetts Institute of Technology, 1986.

Deming, W. E. "Notes on Management in a Hospital." Unpublished memorandum, 1987.

Freidson, E. *Profession of Medicine: A Study in the Sociology of Applied Knowledge*. New York: Dodd-Mead, 1970.

Fullam, F. A. "Implementing Patient-Centered Care in an Emergency Room." *Picker/Commonwealth Report*, 1991, *1*, 2–3.

Garvin, D. A. *Managing Quality: The Strategic and Competitive Edge*. New York: Free Press, 1988.

Gitlow, H. S., and Gitlow, S. J. *The Deming Guide to Quality and Competitive Position*. Englewood Cliffs, N.J.: Prentice Hall, 1987.

Goss, M.E.W. "Patterns of Bureaucracy Among Hospital Staff Physicians." In E. Freidson (ed.), *The Hospital in Modern Society*. New York: Free Press, 1963.

Harris, J. E. "The Internal Organization of Hospitals: Some Economic Implications." *Bell Journal of Economics,* 1977, *8,* 467–482.

Imai, M. *Kaizen: The Key to Japan's Competitive Success.* New York: Random House, 1986.

Ishikawa, K. *What Is Total Quality Control?* Englewood Cliffs, N.J.: Prentice Hall, 1985.

Johnson, J. "Proactive Executives: Prospering in Tough Times." *Hospitals,* Mar. 20, 1991, pp. 22–27.

Johnsson, J., and Anderson, H. J. "1991 Hospital Turnaround of the Year Contest: Mission, Management, and Margins: Winning Hospitals Tell Their Success Stories." *Hospitals,* July 20, 1991, pp. 22–32.

Juran, J. M. *Managerial Breakthrough.* New York: McGraw-Hill, 1964.

Koeck, C., and Levitt, S. "Continuous Quality Improvement and the Organizational Behavior Literature." Unpublished manuscript, Harvard School of Public Health, 1990.

Koska, M. T. "New Study: More MDs Will Seek Management Jobs." *Hospitals,* Oct. 5, 1991a, pp. 48–50.

Koska, M. T. "Quality Improvement Methods Influence Privileging Process." *Hospitals,* July 5, 1991b, p. 78.

Leebov, W., and Scott, G. *Health Care Managers in Transition: Shifting Roles and Changing Organizations.* San Francisco: Jossey-Bass, 1990.

Levitt, T. *The Marketing Imagination.* New York: Free Press, 1986.

Marszalek-Gaucher, E., and Coffey, R. J. *Transforming Healthcare Organizations: How to Achieve and Sustain Organizational Excellence.* San Francisco: Jossey-Bass, 1990.

Morlock, L. L., Alexander, J. A., and Hunter, H. M. "Formal Relationships Among Governing Boards, CEOs, and Medical Staffs in Independent and System Hospitals." *Medical Care,* 1985, *23,* 1193–1213.

Pallarito, K. "Teaching Hospitals, Universities Part Ways." *Modern Healthcare,* Dec. 17, 1990, p. 43.

Pauly, M., and Redisch, M. "The Not-for-Profit Hospital as a Physicians' Cooperative." *American Economic Review,* 1973, *63,* 87–99.

Schein, E. H. *Organizational Culture and Leadership: A Dynamic View*. San Francisco: Jossey-Bass, 1985.

Schlesinger, L. A., and Heskett, J. L. "The Service-Driven Service Company." *Harvard Business Review*, 1991, *69*, 71–81.

Senge, P. M. *The Fifth Discipline: The Art and Practice of the Learning Organization*. New York: Doubleday Currency, 1990.

Shortell, S. M., and others. "Organizational Assessment in Intensive Care Units: Construct Development, Reliability, and Validity of the ICU Nurse-Physician Questionnaire." *Medical Care*, 1991, *29*(8), 709–726.

Slomski, A. J. "Hospitals Wield a Heavy Club Against High-Cost Doctors." *Medical Economics*, 1991, *68*, 56–69.

Steiber, S. R. "How Consumers Perceive Health Care Quality." *Hospitals*, Apr. 5, 1988, p. 84.

"TQM Likely to Change Focus of Physician Privileging Process." *QI/TQM*, 1991, *1*, 49–51.

Wagner, M. "Managing Diversity." *Modern Healthcare*, Sept. 30, 1991, 24–29.

11

Promoting the Doctor's Involvement in Care

Thomas L. Delbanco

On our site visits to hospitals eager to improve the patient-centered quality of their care, both doctors and hospital administrators often reported that doctors were not very involved in efforts to assess and change care. Doctors seemed left out of the central decision-making process—apparently either by their own choice or at the choice of the hospital administration. Even in hospitals espousing principles of continuous quality improvement or participatory management, doctors were rarely involved actively in efforts to improve the patient's experience. When discussing this phenomenon with doctors, we found them exasperated. At times they felt that hospital managers and nurses were consciously excluding the doctor as they addressed "clinical" issues more properly within the doctor's sphere of responsibility. In other cases, they said simply that they face so many overwhelming constraints and administrative hassles that they had neither the energy nor the time to tackle the issues we address in this book.

Patients regard doctors with an extraordinary range of emotion. Each—respect, fear, awe, mistrust, confidence, apprehension, and myriad others—mingles and, at times, dominates. Patients may view their doctors both as individuals, separate and distinct from hospitals, or as part of the fabric of the hospital. They may see them as captains of the ship, or as equal and, at times subordinate, members of a health team. They may view them as the primary caregiver, or as an expert consultant to be seen once and never again. And the patient's view of doctors is colored both by individual anecdote and by aggregate impression. As one hospitalized patient pointed out, "I didn't have a whole lot to occupy my mind sitting in the hospital. I really didn't. So I sort of watched, and I watched real hard. And I observed phenomenal differences across the board, just in the way they, the doctors, treat individuals."

The findings in our national survey point clearly to some of these phenomena and the way hospitalization brings them into sharp focus. Patients watch what is going on closely. More than 10 percent noted doctors talking in front of them as if they were not there. More than 15 percent felt no single doctor was in charge of their care. More than a quarter reported that doctors spent less than five minutes with them preparing them for discharge from the hospital and discussing their medical regimen and other activities to pursue at home. As the writer and editor Anatole Broyard observed, patients are not the only ones shortchanged by this clinical distance: "A doctor's job would be so much more interesting and satisfying if he would occasionally let himself plunge into the patient, if he could lose his own fear of falling" (1990, p. 33).

Doctors have enormous influence on each of the dimensions of patient-centered care. They are virtually certain to affect a hospitalized patient's experience in every dimension. Here, we explore the role doctors play "through the patient's eyes" and propose strategies to involve doctors more actively in improving the patient's experience with hospital care.

How Doctors Think About Patients, Hospitals, and Their Practices

To consider how to involve doctors more actively in the dimensions of care we found so important to patients, we must focus first on several attributes of doctors as a group. I write from the perspective of a general internist who has been active in practice, education, and research for more than twenty years. Many of the impressions that follow derive from that experience, amplified by visits to hospitals and doctors scattered through the United States.

Doctors' view of the hospital is changing. In the past, doctors saw the hospital as a hotel serving both them and their patients. Hospitals were not in the business of delivering care as such. Rather, they catered to two customers: doctor and patient. In the late 1960s and early 1970s, a dramatic shift occurred. Hospitals began hiring doctors to work full time on their wards and in their clinics. With academic health centers taking the lead, the emphasis was first on specialists who worked hard to gain referrals from community-based doctors. In the 1970s, hospitals also began to deploy salaried doctors as primary caregivers; they were based both at the hospital and in nearby practices sponsored and financially supported by the hospital. Thus, depending on where they practiced and how they were supported, doctors began to view hospitals either as competitors or as their employers. Conversely, hospitals view some doctors (and their patients) as customers to be wooed and attracted. They see others as employees whose allegiance is complicated by pride in professional autonomy. Doctors in teaching hospitals encounter a special problem: the complex demands of several masters, including medical schools, practice plans, and outside funding agencies. The president of a prominent teaching hospital notes cryptically that "professors are brought on board primarily to follow their noses rather than the corporate mission."

Doctors believe they are "patient centered." While doctors may not rush to follow hospital administrators, they are clearly eager to please their patients. The suggestion that they may not always be optimally "patient centered" is likely to raise hackles. Doctors, whether in primary care or specialty practices, are convinced that they respond directly and effectively to their patients' needs. And if they recognize difficulty in doing so, they are apt to point to interference from administrative or bureaucratic obstacles.

Doctors worry about the doctor-patient relationship. For many reasons, doctors today bemoan the increasing fragility of the doctor-patient relationship. The forces that threaten a strong and meaningful bond are many. Among them are limited time to establish and maintain the relationship, technology encroaching on and replacing personal interactions, the litigious society, a "comparison shopping" approach to seeking services that more and more characterizes today's customer (or patient), and economic constraints

and barriers that require uncomfortable, explicit discussion between the doctor and patient.

Doctors' roles are shifting. Today, doctors often find themselves taking roles very different from those they expected. O'Connor (1992) has suggested an analogy from sports, with the individ-
ualistic baseball player becoming first a football quarterback and
now, in more recent years, a basketball player sharing with the
patients the pursuit of health care. As this implies, the role many
patients take has shifted, as they become more active in managing
their care. They choose their doctors after comparison shopping,
question their doctors' judgments and seek second opinions, and
view doctors as members of the patient's team who hold special
expertise but are by no means entitled to call all the shots.

Doctors' image is faltering. While patients' attitudes toward
their own doctors remain positive on the whole, public opinion
about doctors in general has plummeted (Blendon, 1988). The
causes of the profession's fall from grace are multiple: greater public
consciousness of the fallibility of medical science; worry and anger
about paternalism, arrogance, out-of-pocket expense, and doctors'
incomes; widely publicized stories of medical negligence, injury,
and fraudulent behavior; and defensive postures by doctors as fee
payment protocols are revised and debate about costs, access, and
the organization of care intensifies. Whatever one believes about the
merits or causes of the changed perceptions, one thing is certain:
doctors are very unhappy about their tarnished public image.

Doctors worry about attracting and retaining patients. Given
the rapid shifts in practice arrangements, payment mechanisms,
and patterns of care, doctors are understandably anxious about their
practices. Whether in fee-for-service, prepaid, individual, group, or
hospital-based practice, doctors find their patients entering and
leaving their practices at unheard-of speed. The reasons are many:
shifting populations, changing insurance coverage, both employer
and individual patient preferences, and changes in the distribution
of health professional manpower. Perhaps the clearest indicator of
doctors' concerns is the rapid proliferation of aggressive marketing
strategies directed at both patients and third-party payers. As one
cardiologist exclaimed, when considering the potential impact of
asking his patients to report on the quality of his practice, "Do you

know what's important about this? *Marketing*, that's what's important! If I let my community know I'm doing a good job with my patients, I'll get more patients. And that's dynamite!"

Doctors like data. From their earliest days of medical education, doctors hear about the importance of making decisions by drawing on data rather than on clinical impression. Medical educators and clinical investigators—the principal role models for the student and young doctor—extol the virtue of the scientific method for evaluating diagnostic methods and therapies. Their mentors deride anecdote and trumpet the virtue of the controlled trial and statistical significance. They urge their students to gather and analyze data. While some have questioned the practitioner's actual dependence on data in making decisions (Avorn, Chen, and Hartley, 1982; Avorn and Soumerai, 1983), doctor rhetoric certainly claims they depend heavily on the "facts."

Doctors thrive on specifics rather than generalizations. Closely related to their interest in data, doctors would rather respond to facts than to others' judgments. They learn little from and are unimpressed by the satisfaction surveys many hospitals conduct. They question their validity and bemoan their lack of specificity. Doctors like material that moves beyond generalization and focuses on discrete events. They find that the data generated by satisfaction surveys are not actionable; they do not point toward a specific response. Practitioners might be concerned, for example, to learn that 25 percent of their patients are "dissatisfied" with their care, but that finding does little to point doctors in a direction that might counteract such an evaluation.

Doctors would rather listen to their patients than to others. It is a truism among hospital administrators, nurses, and other health workers that doctors would rather talk than listen. Many doctors are superb speakers; as one administrator pointed out, "They live with their mouths." But doctors' willingness to listen draws less praise. While patients share others' distress at this attribute, they are apt to win in a competition occurring during the doctor's increasingly busy day. Among the various contenders for the doctor's ear, patients are those most likely to gain the doctor's attention.

Doctors resist quality assurance programs conducted by peers and other health workers. Quality assurance programs addressing clinical competence have a troubled history. Close colleagues hesitate to find fault, and doctors greet with suspicion others who pass judgment. Those reviewed often adopt defensive postures hardly conducive to positive motivation and self-examination—ingredients vital for improved performance. And the costs associated with quality assurance programs that search for those who perform poorly can be considerable. It is not always easy to demonstrate benefits justifying these costs (Berwick, 1989).

Doctors depend heavily on hospital staff. Doctors know that their patients' experience with hospital care is determined in large part by the skill, motivation, and energy of hospital staff. As we discuss throughout this book, these elements affect both the technical and interpersonal elements of care. When hospital staff offer first-class care, the patient often rewards the doctor. Conversely, when care proves flawed, doctors may reap the blame.

Doctors often depend on house staff. Nearly one in every five hospitals in the United States has postgraduate residency or fellowship education programs, according to the Association of American Medical Colleges (information obtained by telephone in Oct. 1992), and an even higher proportion of hospital beds hold patients who encounter house staff during their hospital stay. House staff are often at least as important to hospitalized patients as the attending doctors. Patients may view the house staff as delegates of the doctor who holds prime responsibility, or as the principal doctor in charge. Doctors, both those on a faculty and/or hospital staff, delight in happy reports from patients about house staff. They are equally displeased to learn from their patients that not all has gone well with a patient–house officer interaction.

Doctors are frustrated by poor patient adherence to medical regimens. Doctors find little reward in patients who do not adhere to medical regimens and appear unable to pursue a rational course in managing their illness. On the other hand, they are generally delighted by the patient (and family) eager to follow the doctor's prescriptions and suggestions. Similarly, patients are puzzled by and mistrust the doctor whose suggestions seem out of place. They are more likely to comply with counsel that makes sense to their particular circumstance. In recent years, controlled trials have confirmed what intuitively makes sense: understanding where the patient, family, and doctor are "coming from" enhances the optimal management of the patient's illness (Starfield and others, 1981; Carter, Inui, Kukull, and Haigh, 1982; Wartman, Morlock, Malitz, and Palm, 1983; Greenfield, Kaplan, and Ware, 1985; Putnam, Stiles, Jacob, and James, 1985; Brody and others, 1989; Kaplan, Greenfield, and Ware, 1989, 1990; Smith and Hoppe, 1991).

Doctors work long hours . . . and are enjoying them less. Any strategy to involve doctors more actively in addressing the interpersonal elements of care has to take into account the fact that doctors' time is at a premium. According to the American Medical Association, practicing doctors spend an average of nearly fifty hours a week in direct patient care activities (information obtained by telephone in Oct. 1992). Away from the patient, doctors report that the "work of worry" persists. Unread journals fill the office, phone messages pile up, and difficult clinical decisions abound and leave troubled doctors pondering uncertain judgments derived from incomplete information. And today, increasing administrative requirements and demands from third parties and regulators add to the burden and take an enormous toll.

Strategies for Involving Doctors More Actively

In contrast to years past, we learned in our survey that the patient or the doctor is equally likely to choose where a patient is hospitalized. Both are clearly the hospital's customer. From the hospital's perspective, doctors are customers with special attributes, whether or not they are also hospital employees. Similarly, doctors view hospitals as their customers. It does not take long for doctors to learn that both their own comfort and that of their patients is a function of the nature of the doctor-hospital relationship. In recent years, hospitals have marketed their virtues to doctors primarily by touting technological strengths, both those available and those anticipated. To attract both primary care doctors and patients, hospitals extol the quality of their imaging devices and specialty services. Similarly, to invite specialty doctors, hospitals again highlight their technologies. However, the latest biomedical technologies have become so widely dispersed that soon they will provide little market edge. Hospitals will find them necessary but not sufficient to attract doctors and their patients. In the future, the ability of hospitals to care, in the broadest context, may make the difference between full or empty beds and clinics.

As we turn now to strategies for involving doctors more actively in the dimensions of care we are highlighting, we will base them on the attributes outlined above. We suggest that each strategy can form the foundation for initiatives that bring doctors closer to their patients and to the hospitals on which both—doctor and patient—depend. Each effort should recognize the special needs of the doctor. To involve them actively, one has to recall a basic rule for promoting change in human behavior: the doctor will pose and try to answer the classic question: "What's in it for me?"

The central thesis of what follows has two components: (1) a clear and continuous focus on the hospitalized patient's experience with illness will interest doctors; (2) doctors will join in efforts to improve the quality of care if hospital staff invite them to work on difficult problems in an active and collaborative way. Hospitals might try some of the suggestions that follow.

Use focus groups of patients to show doctors what patients say. Drawing on the observation that doctors would rather listen to patients than to hospital personnel, some hospitals have been pleased with the response of doctors to commentary by patients who join in focus groups to discuss their hospital experience. The discussion can cover broad areas of interest or target discrete dimensions of care. The insights gained often stimulate productive response. Consider the following suggestion from a patient: "If they had told me what I *could* do, that would have been helpful. I've felt so vulnerable that I think I've been a little timid to do things. There wasn't much I could do, but I wasn't told what I could do, and it might have been encouraging." As observers, patients bring a broad perspective. As third parties, their commentary can help break the "we-they" impasse that springs up all too often between doctors and other hospital workers. The commentary on quality that patients offer may be much more acceptable to the doctor than the suggestions of doctor colleagues or other health workers.

The leaders of the focus groups of patients should be carefully trained in the techniques shown to foster success in such efforts. They must work impartially to generate substantive and constructive commentary. They should invite patients drawn at random, compensate them for their time, and avoid the "professional patient" who is less flexible and arrives with a relatively programmed agenda. One-way mirrors and audiotape and videotape recordings help preserve the immediacy and increase the impact of the meetings.

Convene focus groups of doctors. Just as doctors are not always sensitive to issues other hospital workers face, so too can those who work with doctors learn from listening to frank interchange among doctors. Led by trained facilitators, free-floating or categorical discussions by focus groups of doctors can foster mutual understanding. Asking nurses, social workers, administrators, and support personnel to listen to and review the issues raised by doctors can be the first step in initiating constructive dialogue and change. For example, watching a group of doctors talk over the clinical implications of legislation mandating discussion of advance directives may give other ward personnel helpful insights into issues doctors confront.

Challenge doctors to solve difficult problems. From their earliest days in school, students who end up choosing medicine as a career love to solve difficult problems. They are prototypical high achievers, used to rising to the head of the class. For such individuals, the tougher the problems, the more they enjoy tackling them. How can redundancy in laboratory testing be decreased? How can hospital personnel best avoid dangerous contact with contaminated fluids? The prospect of solving problems for which other efforts have failed brings particular satisfaction. As one hospital administrator put it, "Particularly when I work with doctors, I pose problems as a challenge. Doctors invariably rise to the bait."

Give doctors aggregate data about their own patients. While focus groups of patients generate rich anecdotes, aggregate data from patients drawn at random can be a powerful stimulus to self-examination by doctors. In contrast to their feelings about general ratings of satisfaction, doctors will appreciate their patients' reports about discrete events in their care. A survey that tells the doctor that "25 percent of your patients report that they were not told what they could or could not do at home after leaving your office" helps steer the practitioner toward a specific, corrective action. Such reports serve as screening tests, showing doctors areas of care they need to examine and improve (Delbanco, 1992). Most important, these data come from patients themselves, not from colleagues or other health workers peering over the doctor's shoulder. And while patients' reports may differ from what actually takes place, their perceptions remain important. As one senior clinician put it, pondering the value of reports from patients, "Even if I spent time explaining what I want my patient to watch out for, the fact that she didn't remember my doing so means I have to communicate with her differently. It doesn't help to know I did something. What's important is that I didn't get my point across."

Data can have a powerful impact on doctors, and modest but compelling numbers may rapidly initiate change. Many doctors, for example, address patients by their first name, without inquiring first about their preferences. In one hospital, a doctor surveyed patients and documented a variety of responses to this aspect of care. Feedback to colleagues led some to change their habits quickly.

Similarly, two findings in our survey moved a doctor in one hospital to change his behavior. He learned that those acutely ill patients in his hospital who were chronically in poor health encountered more problems with their care than did those generally in good health. He learned further that many of these sick patients recalled spending less than five minutes with a doctor in preparation for discharge. In response, the doctor changed behavior. Concentrating in particular on his patients with chronic illness, he spent more time with them on the day of discharge, addressing in detail what they might or might not do once back home. While this effort led him to spend some extra time on the hospital wards, he believes the net impact has been to save time. Indeed, he appears delighted by his impression that he has decreased morbidity in several of his patients and may well have prevented early readmission for some. He receives fewer phone calls from patients seeking clarification after they return home. He was struck in particular by a patient with renal failure and recurrent electrolyte imbalance leading to hospitalization three times in six months. A more extended discussion at his last discharge revealed relatively simple misconceptions about both his diet and medicines. At the time of writing, the patient has done well at home for more than eight months.

Patient and doctor alike hope to interact in the context of a profoundly caring profession. Gathering organized critiques from those they serve is a dramatic expression of doctors' interest in self-improvement. Asking patients to "help me do better" is a striking way to show that the doctor cares. And again, doctors are more likely to accept criticism and advice from their patients than from others.

Document and develop educational programs about patient-centered care. Few would argue with the notion that those who affect the patient's experience with illness should be humane and caring. Yet such exhortation may not be enough to stimulate doctors to change behavior. Doctors must convince themselves that the dimensions of care addressed in the preceding chapters are more than "frills" that pale in comparison with the biomedical needs of patients.

As interest in clinical epidemiological and health services research grows, data suggest increasingly that the patient's experience with illness affects both the process and the outcome of care. The preceding chapters richly document these findings, but many of the relevant studies appear in journals and books that practitioners are unlikely to read. Clinical reviews, annotated bibliographies, and other methods of continuing education may help inform doctors. Hospitals should take every opportunity to disseminate and emphasize new findings in this area of clinical investigation.

Encourage doctors and patients to improve the way they communicate. Whether for humane and caring reasons or in response to public concern over impersonal care, medical educators—and even certifying boards—pay far more attention today to developing and evaluating the interpersonal skills of doctors than they used to (Brody, 1980; Lipkin, Quill, and Napodano, 1984; Matthews, Sledge, and Lieberman, 1987). Book after book urges patients to address doctors directly and openly. And scholars work to bridge the gap between the clinical language of the practitioner and the patient's language of subjective feeling (Arnold, Forrow, and Barker, 1992; Cassell, 1985; Lipkin, Quill, and Napodano, 1984; Stoeckle, 1987; Donnelly, 1986; Smith and Hoppe, 1991; Kass, 1990; Candib, 1987).

Studies evaluating the clinical impact of the doctor-patient relationship suggest that sharing of responsibility affects clinical outcomes favorably. Greenfield and colleagues (1988) found that teaching patients to be more aggressive in their interactions with doctors leads to better control of blood sugar in diabetics and contributes to improved levels of blood pressure in hypertensive patients. These investigators are now taking the next step, turning their efforts toward helping doctors deal less defensively and more effectively with patients who take a more active role than in the past.

Encourage doctors and patients to review the patient as a unique individual. Sacks (1983, p. 205) reminds both doctor and patient that "there is nothing alive which is not individual: our health is ours; our reactions are ours—no less than our minds or our faces. Our health, diseases, and reactions cannot be understood in vitro, in themselves; they can only be understood with reference to us, as expressions of our nature, our living."

As doctors and patients discuss the seven dimensions of care we describe, it is helpful to establish a framework that promotes systematic review and clearly establishes the unique attributes of the individual patient. Matthews and Feinstein (1988) and Delbanco (1992) suggest that an orderly approach to the dimensions can constitute a "patient's review" that is, in some respects, analogous to the traditional "review of systems" doctors initiate when first evaluating in depth the biomedical components of a patient's illness. In contrast to the traditional review, which is orchestrated and conducted by the doctor, a "patient's review" that makes explicit the patient's desires, apprehensions, and uncertainties often results in dialogue that promotes sharing of responsibility. While such review takes time, it will pay off in establishing or strengthening the doctor-patient relationship. It need not be completed during a single encounter; the doctor and patient can weave it into their ongoing interactions. It helps tailor care to the individual patient, forcing the doctor and patient to make explicit what often has beeen implicit. And as doctor and patient confront and express individual preferences and values, they are more likely to explore a range of options, including nontraditional, alternative therapies. Such review pushes both to expand horizons.

When and how might doctors learn to use such a framework for addressing clinically important components of the patient's illness? Medical educators can incorporate it into the medical school and postgraduate curriculum. It provides a context during the preclinical years for studying cultural, ethnic, and socioeconomic forces that influence how patients experience and manage illness. And during clinical teaching, just as faculty query students and residents about physical signs and symptoms, they can ask about patients' values, preferences, knowledge, and support systems. Matthews, Sledge, and Lieberman (1987) and Brody (1980) have also taken a next step by asking patients themselves for feedback about how students perform.

The idea of asking patients for review and critique can help both the doctor and the patient. One patient, reflecting on his operation for a life-threatening malignancy, noted, "You know, for the surgeon, it was a pretty routine matter. For me, it was one of the major events in my life. I would have liked to be debriefed once it was all over. It would have helped me put things into place, and it might have helped him too. Just five or ten minutes of reflection together would have meant a lot."

Encourage doctors to teach the systematic assessment of patients and their experience to staff. The self-interest of attending doctors should encourage them to enhance relationships between house staff and patients. In settings where house officers and medical students affect patients' experience with hospital care, attending doctors can benefit from teaching their younger partners to pay systematic attention to the dimensions of care that patients consider important. If one accepts the assumption that both the biomedical and subjective, experiential aspects of care affect the outcome, for the patient, attending doctors—as noted above—can address both during teaching rounds. Students and house staff enjoy the variety of discussion that such a broader perspective engenders, and teaching at the bedside takes on greater meaning as the doctor, students, and patient consider together the patient's illness. The patient frequently joins actively in the teaching process, enlivening and clarifying the history and describing the impact of illness from his unique perspective.

In our visits to hospitals with postgraduate training programs, we encountered some examples in which the principal teachers paid considerable attention to developing the interpersonal skills of their students, house staff, and younger faculty. Both the trainees and patients appeared to benefit directly from these efforts. In one urban teaching hospital with severely constrained nursing and support services, patients reported a very positive experience with hospitalization. There, house staff participated in an active program stressing interpersonal skills, and it is likely that this emphasis led to favorable reports from the patients surveyed. House staff felt closely supported by senior faculty and exhibited remarkable esprit, although support services were far fewer than in other hospitals with both dispirited house staff and patients.

Ask patients to teach. There is growing interest in sensitizing health workers to the experience of others who work with them. Hospitals ask senior managers to be "nurse for a day," or "housekeeper for a day." Indeed, the idea of being "patient for a day" is also gaining currency, with some residency programs admitting new trainees to the hospital with factitious illness under a fictitious name.

Similarly, role play among health professionals, among professionals and actors playing patients, or among professionals and volunteering patients can be productive and enjoyable for all concerned. Asking patients to teach brings a wealth of information to the classroom, ward, or clinic; the experience of illness springs into sharp relief for all kinds of students—whether hospital presidents or first-year medical students. Perhaps most important, it elevates the patients, reminding all concerned of their special authority.

Assist doctors in trying out and adopting new ancillary tech-

niques. Several ancillary methods can help doctors and patients focus on the dimensions of care more easily. In some instances, they involve widely available, inexpensive devices. In others, they are early examples of rapidly evolving new technologies.

- *Recording pivotal conversations with patients (and families).* Several doctors and their patients have found it useful to record important conversations. As a noted health professional pointed out, "When my mother became very sick, the whole family assembled to hear the bad news and get advice from the doctor. My brother and sister also have doctoral degrees, but when we got home and began to discuss what the doctor had said, we realized we each remembered a totally different conversation."

  An oncologist we encountered has a tape recorder in each of his office examining rooms and brings along a portable one to the bedside when rounding in the hospital. When conveying important new information to patients or family members, he records the conversation and hands over the recording. He finds that the information it contains will later reach ears far more receptive and understanding than in the anxiety-filled setting of the doctor's office or hospital room.

- *Forwarding written summaries of important doctor-patient interactions.* While or shortly after talking with patients (and families), some doctors find it helpful to dictate notes summarizing important discussions or advice. They report that such letters clarify, remind, and reinforce. A controlled trial demonstrated that patients are grateful for the chance to review and digest what their doctor describes and advises (Damian and Tattersall, 1991). For the doctors, too, such letters serve as helpful records and reminders.

- *Providing patients and families with educational materials.* With the doctor's time so scarce, material that amplifies and complements advice that doctors offer can be helpful to doctor and patient alike. Written educational materials are widely available. With rapidly proliferating computer technologies, doctors can personalize them to document an individual patient's illness. Educational programs that address specific diseases or procedures are also available on audiotape and video-tape. Now, laser discs and interactive television programs also invite patients to take an active role in managing illness. While doctors find such aids important, most have little time to seek them out, separate the wheat from the chaff, and deploy them in a way that makes them easily available to their patients. Hospital staff can help with these efforts, and the interchange can quietly strengthen relations among doctors, staff, and patients.

• *Using automated patient records that free doctors from routine tasks and help enrich the doctor-patient relationship.* Doctors want to move beyond repetition and routine. While compulsive review of facts and contingencies is the hallmark of the first-class doctor, it can also be time consuming and boring. Computers can help doctors complete routine tasks, and hospitals can offer such technologies and teach doctors to use them. The doctor can use the time saved to establish and promote a strong and rewarding doctor-patient relationship.

Several hospitals are close to using a paperless patient record. Compared to the traditional paper record, the doctor may need as much, or more, time initially to generate a computerized record. But in subsequent visits or encounters on the ward, the flexibility and efficiency of an automated record are extraordinary.

The patient record, traditionally controlled by the doctor, has the potential both to reflect and promote a shared doctor-patient relationship. While early experiments that evaluated the impact of having both doctor and patient write in the record proved awkward and inefficient (Fischbach, Sionelo-Bayog, Needle, and Delbanco, 1980), the automated record provides an exciting opportunity for the future. Patients and their families can learn both to review the doctor's impressions and counsel and to enter their own observations and suggestions. The computer provides a framework that encourages structured, organized input from both the doctor and the patient. It can also accept free text, with anecdote that highlights the unique circumstance.

Reward and honor doctors for outstanding performance. Hospitals commonly provide reward and recognition programs that highlight outstanding performance by their employees. These programs have centered primarily on length of service and technical achievement, but some are now recognizing efforts to improve quality, including the quality of the interpersonal aspects of patient care. Doctors have played a relatively minor role in these programs. In part, this derives from their complex and often ambiguous relationship to the hospital. On the other hand, professional societies understand that doctors appreciate recognition, and hospitals might draw on their example. Recognition in employee newsletters and awards for outstanding achievement in the personal elements of care can mean a lot to doctors. Testimonials from patients can have striking impact. Those that describe specific actions have much more impact than does general praise and may in themselves prove educational. For example, in a letter to the doctors in a large practice, a patient noted, "She is a young doctor, and she took time to get to know what I am all about. I had never felt free before to share my fears with a doctor. Just the fact that she understood what I was afraid of made an incredible difference. It helped me keep myself together through an awful illness, and I think today it is helping me recover more quickly." There is little that could mean more to a doctor.

Summary

Doctors affect each element of care that patients believe important. Today there are enormous forces, some clearly external and some self-imposed, that distance doctors from their patients. Doctors know it is in their best interest to draw closer to their patients. Hospitals need to understand what it is to be a doctor. They can draw on such understanding to help doctors improve the way they offer and deliver care. Strategies that give doctors feedback about their own patients' experiences and that use patients as teachers are likely to be more effective than quality assurance programs that search out individual poor performers.

References

Arnold, R., Forrow, L., and Barker, L. R. "Medical Ethics and Patient-Physician Communication." In M. Lipkin, S. M. Putnam, and A. Lazare (eds.), *The Medical Interview*. New York: Springer-Verlag, 1992.

Avorn, J., Chen, M., and Hartley, R. "Scientific Versus Commercial Sources of Influence on the Prescribing Behavior of Physicians." *American Journal of Medicine*, 1982, *73*, 4-8.

Avorn, J., and Soumerai, S. B. "Improving Drug-Therapy Decisions Through Educational Outreach: A Randomized Controlled Trial of Academically Based 'Detailing.'" *New England Journal of Medicine*, 1983, *308*, 1457-1463.

Berwick, D. M. "Continuous Improvement as an Ideal in Health Care." *New England Journal of Medicine*, 1989, *320*, 53-56.

Blendon, R. J. "The Public's View of the Future of Health Care." *Journal of the American Medical Association*, 1988, *259*, 3587-3593.

Brody, D. S. "Feedback from Patients as a Means of Teaching the Nontechnological Aspects of Medical Care." *Journal of Medical Education*, 1980, *55*, 34-41.

Brody, D. S., and others. "Patient Perception of Involvement in Medical Care: Relationship to Illness Attitudes and Outcomes." *Journal of General Internal Medicine*, 1989, *4*, 506-511.

Broyard, A. "Doctor, Talk to Me." *New York Times Magazine*, Aug. 26, 1990, p. 33.

Candib, L. M. "What Doctors Tell About Themselves to Patients: Implications for Intimacy and Reciprocity in the Relationship." *Family Medicine*, 1987, *19*, 23-30.

Carter, W. B., Inui, T. S., Kukull, W. A., and Haigh, V. H. "Outcome-Based Doctor-Patient Interaction Analysis. 2: Identifying Effective Provider and Patient Behavior." *Medical Care*, 1982, *20*, 550-566.

Cassell, E. J. *Talking with Patients*. 2 vols. Cambridge, Mass.: M.I.T. Press, 1985.

Damian, D., and Tattersall, M. H. "Letters to Patients: Improving Communication in Cancer Care." *Lancet*, 1991, *338*, 923-925.

Delbanco, T. L. "Enriching the Doctor-Patient Relationship by Inviting the Patient's Perspective." *Annals of Internal Medicine,* 1992, *116,* 414–418.

Donnelly, W. J. "Medical Language as Symptom: Doctor Talk in Teaching Hospitals." *Perspectives in Biological Medicine,* 1986, *30,* 81–94.

Fischbach, R. L., Sionelo-Bayog, A., Needle, A., and Delbanco, T. L. "The Patient and Practitioner as Co-Authors of the Medical Record." *Patient Counseling and Health Education,* 1980, *2,* 1–5.

Greenfield, S., Kaplan, S. H., and Ware, J. E., Jr. "Expanding Patient Involvement in Care: Effects on Patient Outcomes." *Annals of Internal Medicine,* 1985, *102,* 520–528.

Greenfield, S., and others. "Patients' Participation in Medical Care: Effects on Blood Sugar Control and Quality of Life in Diabetes." *Journal of General Internal Medicine,* 1988, *3,* 448–457.

Kaplan, S. H., Greenfield, S., and Ware, J. E., Jr. "Assessing the Effects of Physician-Patient Interaction on the Outcomes of Chronic Disease." *Medical Care,* 1989, *27,* S110–S127.

Kaplan, S. H., Greenfield, S., and Ware, J. E., Jr. "Impact of the Doctor-Patient Relationship on the Outcomes of Chronic Disease." In M. Stewart and D. Boter (eds.), *Communicating with Patients in Medical Practice.* Newbury Park, Calif.: Sage, 1990.

Kass, L. R. "Practicing Ethics: Where's the Action?" *Hastings Center Report,* 1990, *20,* 5–12.

Lipkin, M., Jr., Quill, T. E., and Napodano, R. J. "The Medical Interview: A Core Curriculum for Residents in Internal Medicine." *Annals of Internal Medicine,* 1984, *100,* 277–284.

Matthews, D. A., and Feinstein, A. R. "A Review of Systems for the Personal Aspects of Patient Care." *American Journal of Medical Science,* 1988, *295,* 159–171.

Matthews, D. A., Sledge, W. H., and Lieberman, P. B. "Evaluation of Intern Performance by Medical Inpatients." *American Journal of Medicine,* 1987, *83,* 938–944.

O'Connor, M. "Presentation to Picker/Commonwealth Public Hospital Task Force," given at the meeting of the National Association of Public Hospitals, Glen Cove, N.Y., Feb. 1992.

Putnam, S. M., Stiles, W. B., Jacob, M. C., and James, S. A. "Patient Exposition and Physician Explanation in Initial Medical Interviews and Outcomes of Clinic Visits." *Medical Care*, 1985, *23*, 74–83.

Sacks, O. *Awakenings*. New York: Dutton, 1983.

Smith, R. C., and Hoppe, R. B. "The Patient's Story: Integrating the Patient- and Physician-Centered Approaches to Interviewing." *Annals of Internal Medicine*, 1991, *115*, 470–477.

Starfield, B., and others. "The Influence of Patient-Practitioner Agreement on Outcome of Care." *American Journal of Public Health*, 1981, *71*, 127–131.

Stoeckle, J. D. (ed.). *Encounters Between Patients and Doctors: An Anthology*. Cambridge, Mass.: M.I.T. Press, 1987.

Wartman, S. A., Morlock, L. L., Malitz, F. E., and Palm, E. A. "Patient Understanding and Satisfaction as Predictors of Compliance." *Medical Care*, 1983, *21*, 886–891.

12

Rebuilding Public Trust
and Confidence

Thomas W. Moloney
Barbara Paul

Public esteem for the American medical system is in critical condition. A powerful frustration overwhelms many Americans when they or their family members become seriously ill. The root of their frustration is more than simply financial. It is also deeply personal. The medical system has lost touch with its essential constituency—patients who are seriously ill or seriously worried. It has lost touch with its essential mission—to serve the needs of those patients.

At any given time, most Americans are healthy. They encounter the medical system only occasionally, through routine checkups and maintenance, processes usually provoking no more anxiety than general dental care. But when serious illness strikes, patients often experience it as an assault on identity and sense of self (Silberman, 1991). It leaves no aspect of life untouched: "Your relationships, your work, your sense of who you are and who you might become, your sense of what life is and ought to be—these all change, and the change is terrifying" (Frank, 1991, p. 6).

Both seriously ill and seriously worried patients can experience powerful sensations and dreaded fears, but they often do not know how to interpret them. They crave information, guidance, and reassurance. They want to know what medicine can do and what they can do for themselves to make the best of whatever their new reality is to be. Even more, they hope for restoration: treatment

280

that will relieve pain, restore their ability to work and function, and restore their senses, their outlook, and their sexuality.

Meanwhile, modern medicine too often behaves as if caring for such human needs is beyond its purpose and beyond the job of its scientifically trained personnel. Medical education stresses pathophysiological process to the exclusion of the social, personal, and even functional dimensions of health and illness. Residency training teaches diagnosis by biotechnical methods, rendering interpersonal skills and human performance measures anachronistic. Modern medicine's allegiance to the pathophysiological pursuit of disease has led practitioners further and further from patients' experiences of illness. Medical financing has followed suit: it so favors the biotechnical aspects of care that the implicit message to professionals is, "Deal with your patients' concerns on your own time."

Leading physicians have warned for over half a century against the widening gulf between the concerns that patients and their families have about serious illness and the preoccupation of medicine with the investigation of disease (McDermott, 1981; Peabody, 1927). Now, for the first time, a new science of patient care promises to bring this disjuncture into alignment. Developing rapidly are techniques to measure with precision how patients experience the process and outcomes of the medical care they receive. Applications of those techniques promise to help medical professionals and institutions reshape the goals and processes of care to better meet patients' needs and help patients achieve a higher quality of life, along a broader range of dimensions.

This chapter examines the potential of this emerging science to bridge the gulf between patients and practitioners and rebuild public trust and confidence in medicine. Discussed first are the changes that have led to the current crisis of public confidence and why restoring public faith is crucial to the medical system's future effectiveness. Second, the chapter looks at broad social, demographic, and technological forces that are fueling a growing demand for a more patient-responsive system. Third, it illustrates major areas of research that have produced breakthroughs that will facilitate greater attention to patients' needs and concerns. The chapter concludes with a vision of the potential benefits that a new era of patient-centered care could bring.

The Erosion of Public Trust and Confidence

The proportion of the American public expressing a great deal of confidence in the leaders of medical institutions and professions has fallen dramatically—from 73 percent in the mid 1960s to 33 percent today (Blendon, 1988). The decline may be part of a broader trend of growing cynicism toward the leaders of major institutions of all types in American society. But it is also rooted in changes in patients' interactions with and expectations of the medical care system that have emerged as modern medicine evolved over the past forty-five years. Four major changes—involving the increasingly specialized training and pursuits of medical practitioners, the explosive development of information technologies, the rising cost of medical care and changes in its financing, and shifting generational values—have converged to undermine Americans' unquestioning faith in the medical system.

The Shattering of the Osler Tradition

Medical practice in the period immediately after World War II was still very much in the tradition of William Osler, the master clinician of the late nineteenth and early twentieth centuries. Osler's style of medical practice was to establish a personal relationship based on trust and confidence with every patient and to make that relationship an explicit part of the therapeutic process: "Osler described medicine as an art, albeit one based on science. . . . He knew that patients are unique individuals and that often their illnesses develop from the very fabric of their lives. . . . He had a genius at establishing friendships with his patients. . . . He could comfort and inspire patients and give them confidence in their ability to get well. . . . He understood how they felt, and he could share his own feelings. He could elicit trust and confidence" (Wheeler, 1990, p. 1543).

Beginning in the 1950s, however, the increasing specialization of the medical profession shattered the Osler tradition. Physicians became more and more narrowly focused on specific organs of the body. The art of ministering to the whole patient gradually faded in importance. The patient-centered approaches of Osler came to be regarded as quaint and old-fashioned.

Ironically, as clinical work has become more advanced, public disaffection with the medical system has steadily grown. Now, public opinion surveys consistently find that Americans are highly satisfied with the caliber of clinical care they receive and support increased investments in medical science and technology (Blendon, 1988), but they perceive serious shortcomings in the amount of personal attention they receive. Witness the frustration of a patient with breast cancer writing in a recent "My Turn" column of *Newsweek* magazine: "I wanted to be treated as a human being, not just as the owner of a defective breast. . . . The instant some pathologist, whom you've never met, looks through a microscope and delivers a verdict that your tumor is malignant, your life is in the hands of medical professionals, whom in most cases you don't know but you're still supposed to trust" (Kaufman, 1989, p. 10).

Patients' most common complaint is that physicians won't make time to talk with them. In a recent survey by the American Medical Association (Harvey and Shubat, 1991), two-thirds of Americans reported that doctors do not spend enough time with their patients. Tighter physician reimbursement is usually considered the culprit. It squeezes time with patients out of the doctor's ever-busier day. Physicians wind up spending less time each year with each patient in order to maintain their incomes. Yet the lack of time spent is also a problem in prepaid group practices, where the economic pinch is not so direct. So there may be more than economic determinism to this story. The lack of time made available may stem from the medical profession's drifting away from the patient-centered practices of William Osler. It may be a manifestation of the difference between the practitioner's focus on the treatment of disease and the patient's longing to discuss the illness.

The End of the Era of Clinical Innocence

Patients' faith in the medical profession has also been challenged by the increasingly sophisticated capabilities and applications of information technologies. The computer has made it feasible to collect and analyze vast quantities of clinical information and to understand, with increasing precision, the extent of scientific uncertainty, the lack of standardization in medical care, and the magnitude of variations in practitioners' skill levels and in the outcomes of care. In short, the computer has put an end to the age of clinical innocence and unchallenged faith in medical progress that flourished in the post–World War II period.

In its place is a new era of patient information. Today's newspaper reader may have more exposure to clinical epidemiology than the average physician forty years ago. For example, a recent report in the *Wall Street Journal* included a chart listing all Pittsburgh-area hospitals by name and displaying each hospital's mortality and morbidity rates by procedure, along with average charges. The report concluded: "For the first time, consumers . . . can compare hospitals on price and performance, much as people compare mileage ratings, service records, and sticker prices when they shop for cars. The implications for the nation's medical care system are huge" (Winslow, 1990, p. B1).

Employers have already begun to disseminate such information directly to employees. Displayed on the company bulletin board of the Hershey Food Corporation, for instance, are comparisons of the costs and outcomes of normal childbirth at fifteen area hospitals.

Patients' Increasing Share of Costs

Beginning in the mid 1940s, American patients and their families were gradually relieved of the direct financial burden of medical care. A forty-year era of expansion in the breadth and depth of health insurance opened, first for private patients (through employers, Blue Cross, and commercial insurers) and then for public patients (through Medicare and Medicaid).

That era of expansion ended by 1985. Gone with it were decades in which the real out-of-pocket costs to families declined even as overall health expenditures soared. Beginning in the mid 1980s, the majority of employed insured Americans began to experience a steady erosion in the depth of their insurance coverage and corresponding increases in their out-of-pocket expenses, in the forms of higher premiums, deductibles, and out-of-pocket ceilings. As the cost of care shifts more and more to patients and their families, they are questioning the value they obtain and exerting greater pressure for a medical system that is more responsive to their needs.

Shifting Generational Values

A major shift in the expectations and preferences of patients has occurred as the largest generation in American history, the baby boomers, has come of age. The attitudes and values of the generation that preceded the baby boomers were shaped by the Depression and World War II. They were a generation that embraced authority, security, and conformity. In health care, they tended to respect the medical system and to follow doctors' orders.

In contrast, the formative experiences of the baby boom generation have been the civil rights movement, feminism, the Vietnam War, Watergate, and the information explosion. Baby boomers tend to be less deferential to authority figures and less loyal to institutions. They seek far more information, involvement, control, and choice regarding the services they buy, including medical care, than does the generation that precedes them. They take for granted that there are important variations in the quality and cost of all types of products and services and believe that careful selection brings rewards. As members of the baby boom generation age and become major purchasers of medical services, they are seeking out responsive practitioners far more vigorously and systematically than their predecessors did.

The Stakes of Eroding Public Trust and Confidence

The changes discussed above have led to a sea change in how patients experience medical care and what they expect from it. Public trust and confidence in the ability of the existing system to meet their needs has declined. Left unchecked, that decline could have far-reaching consequences.

Some observers (Lipset, 1983) believe that the degree of public esteem for any industry is the best predictor of the level of public investment in it and of its freedom from regulation—far more indicative than the relative size or rate of growth of past public investments. High public esteem once sustained the considerable public investment and special privileges granted the health care system, including tax exemption and government subsidies for hospital construction, government purchasing of care for the poor, and immunity from tort liability (Stevens, 1989). The future effectiveness of the medical care system may depend more on public confidence and trust in medical professions and institutions than on any other factor (Schroeder, Zones, and Showstack, 1989).

Defenders of the system often point to surveys that claim patients are highly satisfied with their own doctors, even though a substantial portion do not approve of the medical profession (Blendon, 1988). But virtually all ratings of individuals providing personal services are skewed toward high scores. The majority of parents who are highly dissatisfied with the public school system say they are satisfied with their own children's teachers (Gallup, 1988). Similarly, the same patients who hold their own doctors in high regard now consider the medical profession to be one of the primary culprits in the problems that plague the medical care system (Gallup Organization/Blue Cross and Blue Shield, 1990; *Los Angeles Times,* 1990). Frustrated patients and parents alike are prepared to back dramatic "remedies" for the problems of both systems—remedies that may be shortsighted and that their own doctors and teachers would never endorse.

Public confidence and trust in hospitals presents an analogous situation. There has been a marked increase in the public's perception of hospitals as profit-motivated businesses and a corresponding decline in public confidence in the leaders of these institutions. One consequence is that the tax-exempt status of voluntary hospitals is now in jeopardy. Hospitalized patients are uneasy about finding themselves in profit-motivated institutions at a highly vulnerable time of their lives. The dilemma for hospital leaders is how to restore public confidence in their institutions' allegiance to social and scientific missions.

Who will control the future content of medical practice is ultimately at stake as well. Will protocols for determining what services are reimbursable continue to be devised under contracts from insurers and government agencies, without sanction by medical societies? As financial pressures on managed care systems to reduce utilization intensify, the gap between the insurers' and the profession's standards for reimbursable care are likely to widen. Which side the public takes will depend largely on its relative faith and confidence in the parties involved.

Forces for a New Alignment

Regaining public trust and confidence will require the medical profession to reestablish in the public's mind its fundamental commitment to patients. Medical professionals and institutions have always sought to serve patients' needs, but they have tended to rely on physicians to define those needs. What is called for now are systematic efforts to incorporate the patient's perspective.

Forces for change in that direction are recognizable, formidable, and hard at work. Change toward a more patient-centered system will come because millions more aging American families will experience serious illness and insist on it, because researchers are facilitating it, and because medical practitioners and the leaders of medical organizations are beginning to see its rewards. More specifically, substantial change is inevitable for the following reasons.

Growing Numbers of Chronic Care Patients

The frequency and intensity of the problems patients experience with illness are increasing as the American population ages. As the burden of illness stems increasingly from chronic disease, families are seeking practitioners skilled in addressing a broader range of patient experiences, including functional loss, pain, and anxiety. A circumscribed preoccupation with disease as a response from practitioners will be increasingly inappropriate.

Aging Baby Boomers

As discussed earlier, members of the baby boom generation seek out patient-responsive practitioners far more actively than their elders.

Not surprising, the first real changes in health care have come in the services they use first: far greater family accessibility and partici- pation in birthing and pediatric units. The vast majority of this largest generation in American history will enter their forties and fifties during this decade. Their distinctive expectations about their own care, as well as about the care they will choose and manage for their parents, will soon be felt in internal medicine and geriatrics.

Patients' Role in Choosing Providers

Many patients are now actively involved in the choice of medical services themselves. Gone is the traditional reliance on doctors alone to choose hospitals, specialists, and facilities (Christensen and Inguanzo, 1989). In the Picker/Commonwealth survey, half of the patients interviewed said that they or their family—not the doctor— had chosen the hospital. Many patients now even choose a health plan or hospital first and then choose a doctor from among those affiliated. Loyalty to a single provider is not common; many pa- tients report they have switched hospitals or doctors recently or are considering doing so (Cousins, 1985; "Former Patients . . .," 1990).

How Patients Choose

Patients are basing their choices of practitioners and hospitals on factors other than technical quality (Louis Harris and Associates, 1985). The rapid diffusion of medical technology throughout the United States has made it extremely difficult for any hospital to establish a technological edge that is perceptible to patients. Most patients assume that regardless of where they are hospitalized, they will have access to modern facilities, state-of-the-art diagnostic and therapeutic technologies, and a corps of superbly trained specialists. Furthermore, patients are rarely able to distinguish differences in practitioners' abilities to provide complex technical care (Cleary and McNeil, 1988). They are far more likely to focus on differences in providers' readiness and ability to address the range of problems that accompany serious illness than on differences in their technical skills.

New Interest in Patients' Ratings

To judge providers' relative abilities to meet patients' needs, new kinds of information are needed. Patients themselves are often the best source. J. D. Power changed the nature of the automotive marketplace and influenced the design of future cars by making consumer ratings of various aspects of new-model automobiles widely available to the public. Now, vast improvements in information processing technology are making it feasible to publish patients' ratings of the relative ability of competing health care providers to address the full range of problems that severe illness presents. Patients look forward to using their neighbors' ratings in deciding where to seek care in the future. Can the day be far ahead when employers, insurers, consumer groups, or even national periodicals publish surveys of patients' experiences with care received from competing medical plans, at competing hospitals or group practices?

The Picker/Commonwealth Patient-Centered Care survey provides evidence of strong public interest in such information. More than 90 percent of 6,500 recently hospitalized patients who were interviewed said that information about how other patients rate different hospitals should be available to the public. Three-quarters of respondents said that if such information were available, it would influence their choice of hospital.

The Breakthroughs

The major obstacle to putting the patient's experiences of illness at the center of the medical care process has been medicine's steadfast allegiance to the rules of biomedical science. An enduring principle is that the only relevant phenomena are those that can be observed, described, and measured in an objective manner. To be relevant, phenomena have to be describable with quantifiable precision by independent observers at different times (Feinstein, 1967).

But the problems that most concern patients often fail to meet this criterion. How does a scientific practitioner measure and respond to the "severity" of a patient's pain, the "extent" of social functioning, or the "degree" of anxiety? Witness the hesitancy expressed about the quantification of kindness in this recent medical journal article: "Any new chemotherapeutic drug that tripled the survival of patients with incurable cancer would cause great excitement, but we do not know quite how to handle the fact that kindness, emotional support, and optimism have quantitative therapeutic activity" (Wheeler, 1990, p. 1546).

Expanding the scope of medical science requires advances in the measurement of the "soft" phenomena of patients' health and illness. Recent research can claim breakthroughs in a number of areas, including patients' reports of their well-being, the effects of patient control over treatment choices, the role of physician encouragement in the healing process, and aspects of the hospital process that help and hinder recovery.

Measuring Outcomes That Matter to Patients

Recent measurement breakthroughs are enabling researchers and practitioners to obtain and utilize information about the kinds of outcomes that matter most to patients, without violating the basic principles of biomedical science. A team headed by John Ware, Jr., has developed methods to quantify patients' statements about how well they function and how well they feel into objective measurements. The group developed the first assessment tools to provide valid, reliable measures of a range of the problems patients care most about, including functional status, degree of disability, cognitive functioning, emotional health, and social interaction (Tarlov and others, 1989; Stewart and others, 1989; Wells and others, 1989). For the first time, the patient becomes both the recorder and reporter of information now crucial to the diagnosis and treatment processes.

These innovations could transform the ways in which chronic and fatal illnesses are managed. They will expand the boundaries of the scientific approach to disease management to include how well patients function and how well they feel. Once these new measures become widely available, remaining "scientific" will require practitioners to seek information about the broader aspects of their patients' experiences of illness.

Measuring outcomes that matter to patients could also

change the way in which medical care is valued. Measuring quality will require going beyond traditional physiological and clinical indexes of how various body organs respond to treatment. It will entail determining how various treatments affect the quality of life of the individual patient. The patient's experience of illness moves to the center of the care and evaluation processes.

Using the Patient's Perspective in Treatment Choices

Other researchers have moved the valuation of quality even more toward the individual patient's concerns. For example, Wennberg, Mulley, and colleagues observe that for a number of medical conditions, no amount of objective clinical or physiological data is adequate to make an appropriate clinical choice among competing therapies. For conditions such as an enlarged prostate or breast cancer, the decision can be made only by careful reference to a particular patient's unique perceptions and valuations of the likely risks and benefits of alternative therapies (Wennberg and others, 1988; Barry, Mulley, Fowler, and Wennberg, 1988; Fowler and others, 1988). Only with a careful understanding of the patient's values can the physician recommend an appropriate choice of therapy.

This observation suggests a need to better inform patients about their illnesses and the benefits and risks of alternative therapies, as well as a need to develop better methods of patient education. Without assistance, office-based physicians cannot be expected to provide patient education appropriate to understanding the risks and benefits of alternative treatments.

Wennberg and Mulley are developing interactive videodiscs as the patient education technology of the future. The discs use scripts and graphics to convey the nature of an illness and the effects of alternative treatments. They are based on the best clinical research and are tested for patient understanding. If this technology proves successful, video stores throughout the country may one day stock illness-specific educational films. Patients' literacy about their conditions and the caliber and frequency of their participation in selecting treatments could increase dramatically.

Coaching Patients to Improve Their Outcomes

Practitioners' skills in coaching patients may have important, measurable effects on their well-being. Kaplan, Greenfield, and Ware (1989) have demonstrated that coaching patients with chronic illness to become more involved in their care can improve their health, as measured by traditional physiological indices such as blood glucose levels and diastolic blood pressure as well as by improvements in physical functioning. They urge the medical system to recognize the importance of the coaching role by teaching and rewarding practitioners to motivate patients to take steps toward their own recovery; this includes teaching patients self-help skills to aid recovery, coping techniques to minimize the effects of pain or disability, and methods to develop a greater sense of control over functioning. The practitioner's skills as coach will take on greater importance as the burden of illness in the United States shifts increasingly toward chronic diseases, rendering the patient's behavior itself—diet, exercise, life-style changes, and medications—a more crucial part of treatment.

More needs to be known about how well various practitioners' coaching styles work—another crucial yet previously "nonscientific" topic. Medical outcome studies offer an important opportunity to examine which physician styles match best with improved patient functioning and well-being for various types of patients. Such analysis is timely, in view of the decision by the American Board of Internal Medicine that medical residents should demonstrate competence in interpersonal skills as a condition of certification. It could open a "scientific" era of research, education, and training on how to improve physician coaching, as well as patient motivation and compliance.

Improving Patients' Well-Being During the Hospital Process

Researchers and practitioners, determined to develop care processes sensitive to the way patients experience illness, have singled out hospitalization to receive special attention because of its unique trauma-provoking potential. Hospitalization embodies all that is terrorizing about serious illness. On entering a hospital, patients surrender control over their time, privacy, activities, comfort, and clothes. They forgo the reassurance, intimacy, and diversions from worry that the companionship of their family and friends normally provides.

At a most vulnerable time in life, life itself becomes unfamiliar and beyond control, as a series of uniformed strangers take charge of every activity. Patients get interviewed, wheeled, scoped, poked, and processed on whatever shifting schedules they can be slotted into, alongside hundreds of others being hurriedly "worked up" in similar ways. Such events are usually a prelude to far more bewildering treatment and recovery phases. Hospitalization amounts to the gravest form of incarceration most noncriminals ever experience.

The hospitalization process was never designed with the patient in mind. It is instead the residual of thousands of continuous accommodations to the acquisition of new technologies and to the competing demands of the various practitioner groups who command those technologies. Most hospitals compete in a fierce technology-driven race, recruiting the best-trained personnel to provide the latest products, using the most modern equipment. Hospitals have rarely been urged and never rewarded for devising a care process starting from the experiences and concerns of patients. Individual professionals who dedicate their personal attention to the well-being of their patients often do so against tremendous odds, fighting a system with a distinctly different agenda. Hospitals are just beginning to recognize that tomorrow's patients will flock to those hospitals that provide excellent patient care as well as top-notch technical services.

Researchers and practitioners are calling for far more than a public relations campaign or a refurbishing of the hotel-like services hospitals provide. They aim to establish systems for the continuous improvement of hospital practices, based on the careful examination of patients' experiences. They seek to preserve and replicate practices that enhance patients' well-being and to revise practices that contribute to inappropriately high rates of unacceptable patient experiences. The longer-term goal is to enable hospital staffs to incorporate the systematic improvement of patients' experiences into their institutions' systems for monitoring and improving quality and into their professional conception of what good practice requires.

Systematic efforts to understand just how today's hospital practices collide with the patients' needs have just begun. Only recently have survey techniques, applied in other fields for years, been called into service to dissect how patients actually experience the hospitalization process. Doing so was previously considered an impossible task: different patients need different things, and their needs are constantly changing. To circumvent the infinite diversity in patients' preferences, surveyors target patients' actual experiences. They learn the frequency and intensity with which undesirable events occur and positive events are neglected. Previous chapters of this book describe in detail the work of a team led by Thomas L. Delbanco in pinpointing the nature and severity of the problems patients experience during hospitalization.

Such information is only the beginning. Hospitals must then determine which staff groups have the opportunity to improve specific problems, make them aware of the problems, involve them in devising solutions, enlist their cooperation in carrying out new approaches, and provide incentives and reinforcements to help ensure that new behaviors become part of a new standard practice. As the practices highlighted in this book suggest, a patient-centered approach may entail a complete reorganization of hospital practices, including changes in staffing roles and responsibilities, work priorities, and interpersonal styles. Implementing such changes and developing continuous monitoring systems to convey relevant feedback from patients to the staff members who can use it, in a timely fashion, require ingenuity and effort.

The Potential

The groundwork for a major evolution in American medical care is being laid as researchers and practitioners seek ways to better understand and respond to the needs and experiences of seriously ill patients. A new science of patient care is emerging and will work its way into the fabric of the American medical system. Over time, it could bring profound benefits.

It could put the medical care system more squarely in the business of serving the needs of patients with chronic and serious illness. This could change the nature of medical inquiry, leading to vast improvements in physical and social functioning, the reduction of pain, and the relief of anxieties that accompany illness.

It could expand the business of medical care and the pursuits of its practitioners. It could lead, at long last, to a discernibly different role for the generalist practitioner, one in which the patient's reports are crucial diagnostic information and the physician's counsel is a crucial therapeutic tool. It could lead also to the creation of new provider teams, including nurses, psychologists, educators, nutritionists, and physical therapists, as well as generalist physicians.

An expanded concept of the purpose and value of the practitioner-patient interaction could in turn lead the medical payment system to revalue the time practitioners spend with patients. Under an expanded view of medicine, patients become recorders and reporters of their functioning and well-being, partners in the determination of the appropriate course of treatment and partners in their own therapy, carrying through on prescribed life-style changes. Time spent with patients is essential to making these new roles possible. After decades of a technology-dominated reimbursement system, the Physician Payment Review Commission has begun to push the rewards in the direction of more time with patients. Insurers could follow suit, placing greater relative monetary value on time spent with patients.

The emerging science of patient care could spawn a generation of patient-interactive technologies, including educational material on the risks and rewards of treatment options and on self-management of chronic disease, as well as survey information on patients' assessments of competing medical groups, hospitals, and medical care plans. Patient-administered and monitored treatments should also become commonplace: self-administered pain medication in hospitals is only the beginning.

It could also change how medical care is valued. It could usher in a system in which the patient's values regarding risks and rewards are central to determining the "appropriate" course of treatment, one in which a treatment's value is gauged in terms of such "soft" measures as the ability to improve patients' functioning or to relieve pain, anxiety, or depression. This would lead to a vast change in the type of information that is collected and analyzed to assess value. It could limit the use of protocols as the standards of "appropriate" treatment, as patients' particular assessments of risks and benefits become more essential to many treatment decisions.

It could even alter the scope of medical education and the mix of applicants. Medical education for general practitioners of tomorrow may entail far more integration with knowledge from disciplines such as physical therapy, psychology, and sociology. The research methodologies of those disciplines would be integrated toward an expanded notion of the biomedical science paradigm.

Finally, the sum of these changes could restore public esteem for medical professionals and institutions. The extent to which Americans are willing to invest in the medical care system in the future and the relative influence they are willing to grant the medical profession in shaping public policy toward health care may depend more on the level of public trust and confidence, built through a better response to the needs of patients, than on any other factor.

References

Barry, M. J., Mulley, A. G., Jr., Fowler, F. J., and Wennberg, J. E. "Watchful Waiting vs. Immediate Transurethral Resection for Symptomatic Prostatism: The Importance of Patients' Preferences." *Journal of the American Medical Association*, 1988, *259*, 3010–3017.

Blendon, R. J. "The Public's View of the Future of Health Care." *Journal of the American Medical Association*, 1988, *259*, 3587–3593.

Christensen, M., and Inguanzo, J. M. "Smart Consumers Present a Marketing Challenge." *Hospitals*, Aug. 20, 1989, pp. 42–47.

Cleary, P. D., and McNeil, B. J. "Patient Satisfaction as an Indicator of Quality Care." *Inquiry*, 1988, *25*, 25–36.

Cousins, N. "How Patients Appraise Physicians." *New England Journal of Medicine*, 1985, *313*, 1422–1424.

Feinstein, A. R. *Clinical Judgment.* Huntington, N.Y.: Krieger, 1967.

"Former Patients May Not Be as Loyal, Study Shows." *Modern HealthCare,* May 7, 1990, p. 39.

Fowler, F. J., and others. "Symptom Status and Quality of Life Following Prostatectomy." *Journal of the American Medical Association,* 1988, *259,* 3018-3022.

Frank, A. W. *At the Will of the Body.* Boston: Houghton Mifflin, 1991.

Gallup Organization. *The 20th Annual Gallup Poll of the Public's Attitudes Toward the Public Schools.* Princeton, N.J.: Gallup Organization, 1988.

Gallup Organization/Blue Cross and Blue Shield. *Second Opinions: America's Voices and Views on Health Care.* Storrs, Ct.: Roper Center for Public Opinion Research, 1990.

Harvey, L. K., and Shubat, S. C. *Physician and Public Opinion on Health Care Issues.* Chicago: American Medical Association, 1991.

Kaplan, S. H., Greenfield, S., and Ware, J. E., Jr. "Assessing the Effects of Physician-Patient Interactions on the Outcomes of Chronic Disease." *Medical Care,* 1989, *27,* S110-S127.

Kaufman, M. "Cancer: Facts vs. Feelings." *Newsweek,* Apr. 24, 1989, p. 10.

Lipset, M. L. *The Confidence Cap: Business, Labor, and Government in the Public Mind.* New York: Free Press, 1983.

Los Angeles Times. Health Care in the United States. Los Angeles Times Poll #2/2. Storrs, Ct.: Roper Center for Public Opinion Research, 1990.

Louis Harris and Associates. *Americans and Their Doctors.* Survey conducted for Pfizer Pharmaceuticals. New York: Louis Harris and Associates, 1985.

McDermott, W. "Absence of Indicators of the Influence of Its Physicians on a Society's Health." *American Journal of Medicine,* 1981, *70,* 833-843.

Peabody, F. W. "The Care of the Patient." *Journal of the American Medical Association,* 1927, *88,* 877-882.

Schroeder, S. A., Zones, J. S., and Showstack, J. "Academic Medicine as a Public Trust." *Journal of the American Medical Association,* 1989, *262,* 803–812.

Silberman, C. E. "From the Patient's Bed." *Health Management Quarterly,* 1991, *13,* 12–15.

Stevens, R. *In Sickness and in Wealth: American Hospitals in the Twentieth Century.* New York: Basic Books, 1989.

Stewart, A. L., and others. "Functional Status and Well-Being of Patients with Chronic Conditions: Results from the Medical Outcomes Study." *Journal of the American Medical Association,* 1989, *262,* 907–913.

Tarlov, A. R., and others. "The Medical Outcomes Study: An Application of Methods for Monitoring the Results of Medical Care." *Journal of the American Medical Association,* 1989, *262,* 925–930.

Wells, K. B., and others. "The Functioning and Well-Being of Depressed Patients." *Journal of the American Medical Association,* 1989, *262,* 914–919.

Wennberg, J. E., and others. "An Assessment of Prostatectomy for Benign Urinary Tract Obstruction: Geographic Variations and the Evaluation of Medical Care Outcomes." *Journal of the American Medical Association,* 1988, *259,* 3027–3030.

Wheeler, H. B. "Shattuck Lecture: Healing and Heroism." *New England Journal of Medicine,* 1990, *322,* 1546.

Winslow, R. "Data Spur Debate on Hospital Quality." *Wall Street Journal,* May 24, 1990, p. B1.

AFTERWORD

Two things we have learned in the past five years of the Picker/ Commonwealth Program for Patient-Centered Care seem most important to us. First, we have learned that we need to develop systematic, appropriate, and effective ways to ask patients what they need, expect, and experience. And we need to use this information to shape and improve the way we deliver health care. Unless we understand and meet patients' subjective needs, we cannot hope to build confidence and trust in any provider, institution, or health care system. We need to develop this capacity both in *particular*, at the individual level of each patient and each clinical encounter, and in *general*, to understand the aggregate experience of patients within our institutions and systems of care. The appropriateness of any method will depend on its use. We have alluded to some methods in these pages: face-to-face interviews, focus groups, videotaped discussions, and patient surveys. The expertise about such methodologies is much too vast to explore in this volume, drawing as it does on diverse experience in communications, social marketing, and social science research, to name a few of the relevant fields. However, this expertise has rarely been tapped in the service of health care. Health care providers and institutions have been remarkably unsophisticated about methods of eliciting feedback from their patients.

Still, to most of the health care professionals and workers with whom we have talked over the past few years, the concept of "patient-centered care" resonates, widely and harmoniously, with the basic desire to help people that brought them into health care in the first place. Curiously, though, and this is the second thing we have learned: we have discovered not only a lack of familiarity with the methods, but a fundamental and widespread *resistance* to involving patients in planning, designing, or evaluating care. The reason, we believe, is that virtually everyone who works in health care is motivated by genuine humanitarian concern for the sick; almost everyone believes, therefore, that problems must lie elsewhere; and practically no one really wants to listen to, much less invite, a message that may suggest otherwise. The more we solicit and incorporate patients' perspectives, the more each of us, individually, will have to confront our own limitations and the more health care managers and planners will have to find ways to overcome institutional resistance and convert the good intentions of health professionals into a drive for self-examination and improvement.

The task of creating a more humane, equitable, high-quality system of health care ultimately falls to everyone who works in the field. We can do a lot better.

Name Index

SUBJECT INDEX

Sears, part-timers at, 241
Self-care movement, and education, 113–114
Self-help groups, emotional support from, 171–172
Shelby County Health Care Corporation, 251
Significant others. *See* Family
Skagit Valley Hospital and Health Center, education from, 108
Social support. *See* Emotional support
Society for General Internal Medicine, Collaborative Study Group of, 88
South Nassau Communities Hospital, People Activated Toward Health at, 110
Staff: education for, 109–110; information for, 61–63; and physicians, 265, 273
Stanford Medical Center, Arthritis Self-Management Course at, 108
Stanford University, and emotional support, 154–155
Stress, emotional support for coping with, 159–160, 165–167
Summit Medical Center, Cancer Education and Prevention Center at, 106
Support groups, emotional support from, 168–171

T

Tampa General Hospital, GENE-SIS Health Center at, 112
Tennessee Medical School, University of, and change, 253
Texas Children's Hospital, Cystic Fibrosis Program of, 194
Texas in Houston, University of, M. D. Anderson Cancer Center at, 104
Third-party payers, and education, 103, 107
Thomas Jefferson University Hospital, transition from, 208
Transition: attention to, 10–11, 204–223; background on, 204–

206; and community coordination, 217–219; and education, 112; patient view of, 207–211; planning for, 215–217; strategies for, 211–219; suggestions for, 220; summary on, 219
Trinity Hospital: housekeepers at, 66; human resources at, 239
Trust. *See* Public trust and confidence

U

UCLA Medical Center, and family support, 196
United Family Practice, merger with, 114
United Kingdom: communication in, 78; education in, 101
U.S. Army, wellness prescription of, 113
University Hospital, Family Crisis Intervention Program at, 196
Utah Hospital, University of, emotional support from, 167

V

Valley Regional Hospital, and family support, 196
Values: and communication, 83; generational, 285; and preferences and needs, 5–6
Veteran's Hospitals, and emotional support, 160
Virginia, University of, Patient Education Department at, 110
Visitor waiting areas, environment of, 142–144

W

Washoe Medical Center, and family support, 196
Wholistic Health Center, and education, 106–107
Wilson Memorial Hospital, transition from, 213
Winchedon Hospital, closing of, 1–2
Wishard Memorial Hospital, transition from, 213